Thoughts on Chaos in Body and Mind

"*Chaos in Body and Mind* is a vivid and stirring account of Guillain-Barré's ravaging cascade of pain, disability and arduous recovery. Carole Williams' exquisite rendering of not only her illness experience, but her subsequent odyssey through our health care system, is a poignant reminder of the importance of compassion, encouragement, and the preservation of patient dignity as essential elements of the healing process." **Karen Mueller, PT, DPT, PhD, Professor, Program in Physical Therapy, Northern Arizona University, Flagstaff, Arizona**

"This book, written from a very personal perspective, provides critical information to caregivers and families of Guillain-Barré Syndrome victims on the complexity of this rare disease and the need to be responsive to the needs of any patient unable to express his or her needs. Reads like a novel, but informs like a textbook." **Carolyn Roberts, Former Chair American Hospital Association, Green Valley, Arizona**

"At last a book, thoughtfully detailed and well-written, which can prepare both patients and professionals for the long frightening journey Guillain-Barré Syndrome thrusts upon them all." **Ned Yellig, MD, FACP, Raleigh, North Carolina**

"Not only does Carole describe the devastation to her body, but also she gives a vividly detailed picture of her constant struggle with physical and psychological pain as she endures the overwhelming effects of GBS. Truly her mind was trying to survive in total chaos! This book is an informative and challenging read for students and professionals in all mental and health fields." **Dr. Emile Bareng, Psychologist, Kula, Hawaii**

"This very personal account of Carole Williams' long battle helped me to better deal with my own struggle with GBS. It is a must read for all patients and their caregivers affected by this mysterious syndrome." **Robert L. Petrella, DMA, Washington DC**

"The details, descriptive accounts, and emotional impact in Williams' inspirational book should be required reading for everyone in the medical field especially physical and occupational therapists. Patients and their caregivers will laugh and cry their way through this compelling story." **Karl Stoerker, Property Manager, Maui, Hawaii**

"For families struggling with GBS, this book offers valuable insights, hope, wisdom, and even in the midst of suffering, humor and down to earth tips for the patient and loved ones. This honest but hopeful memoir serves as a guide to everyone associated with a GBS patient." **Sylvia White, English teacher and language coach, Raleigh, North Carolina**

"Carole Williams skillfully blends her personal story of Guillain-Barré Syndrome with a lucid explanation of how disruptive this condition can be for patient and family. *Chaos in Body and Mind* is a most important book for both patient and healthcare provider, shedding light on recovery and reclamation." **Dr. Seth Oberst, Doctor of Physical Therapy, Atlanta, GA**

"Gripping from the first page! I highly recommend this book to any patient or family member struggling through a life changing event. Carole's candor and spirit provokes hope for anyone struggling with an injury unseen by the naked eye. This book fosters a change in how we look at disease, rehabilitation and recovery." **Elizabeth Huls PT, DPT, Shepherd Center Acquired Brain Injury Unit, Atlanta, Georgia**

"The Williams' gripping account of their battle with a devastating disease, from first notice that something was wrong through intensity of treatment and rehabilitation, carries powerful messages for doctors, nurses, therapists and counselors. It is an inside recounting of the ultimate level of courage, persistence, and love which are so necessary to overcoming frightening medical uncertainty. The raw emotions and value of positive thinking make this a book everyone should read." **Stephen F. Loebs, Ph.D. Professor Emeritus, Graduate Program in Health Management and Policy, The Ohio State University**

"This book is a must-read for all health care professionals. The Williams use richly expressive detail to document their thoughts and feelings as she confronted physical and rehabilitation challenges during a long-term hospitalization with Guillain-Barré Syndrome. Learning from their journey and the insights they share, will help practitioners become more aware of how their actions affect patients and families." **Sandra Cornett, Ph.D., R.N., Former Patient & Family Education Manager, The Ohio State University Wexner Medical Center, Columbus, Ohio**

"Do not jump ahead in this book! You will want to share Carole's and Stu's experiences as they weave medical messages into an expertly told tale. From the devastating plunge from health to total paralysis, you will follow a well-crafted path to the conclusion of their epic struggle. Gripping tales of the diverse personalities involved in her care read like a Dickens novel. A book with relevance far beyond Guillain-Barré Syndrome." **Bernard Zahren, CEO, Clean Feet Investors, Avon, Connecticut**

CHAOS

IN BODY AND MIND

Our Battle with Guillain-Barré Syndrome

Carole J Williams
with Stuart W Williams

Cover design by Owen Lowery

ISBN: 9781976752490

This book is dedicated to physical and occupational therapists who devote their professional lives to helping people reclaim as much function as possible after a traumatic injury or illness. And particularly to our daughter-in-law, Petra, who taught us this valuable truth.

CONTENTS

Preface

When catastrophic disease strikes, it finds its victims unprepared. They aren't mentally primed to grapple with the complexities of the medical system. Or physically ready to counter the attack on their bodies. And they aren't emotionally geared to handle the rapid and staggeringly chaotic changes to their life's plan which was unfolding, just yesterday, as expected.

Sometimes the advent is slow enough to allow the victim to visit the family doctor, study the symptoms and prognosis, find qualified specialists, and begin treatment. Others give the patient and family no time to do any of these things. Guillain-Barré Syndrome is one of those: a rare and frightening disease that comes stealthily out of nowhere, debilitating its victims with little warning.

Chaos in Body and Mind tells the story of our family's struggle with Guillain-Barré Syndrome from the early twinges of pain that signaled its onset through grueling physical therapy to eventual recovery.

The medical team's approach is critical. In the early stages their decisions set the patient on the course to recovery, but each day is a challenge for them as well as for the patient. Throughout our experience we found many health professionals who knew little about Guillain-Barré Syndrome. Some took extra time to learn what they could about the disease to improve the treatment they were providing. Others seemed to take a fallback position, treating the symptoms they saw each day but never finding creative ways to advance recovery.

Physical and occupational therapists are the most consequential caregivers when battling back from paralysis. Their chosen approach can prompt both physical and psychological improvements throughout this long battle. To us, they were the cornerstone to recovery. Without them, return to a normal life would have been impossible.

For families, who are equally stunned by the rapid onset of Guillain-Barré Syndrome, the mysteries of the disease are more than perplexing. While struggling with early treatment decisions, they also try to find information about the disease and what they can expect as treatment unfolds. Our family found few resources until someone directed us to the Guillain-Barré Syndrome Foundation, the source for a number of pamphlets written in layman's terms, and connection to former patients and family members willing to share their thoughts on how to deal with a long hospitalization and at-home recovery.

We intend this recollection of our journey through a complicated medical system, fighting a rare disease, to help others who face the same monumental challenge. Patients and their families may learn what to expect as they progress through an unknown medical odyssey of their own. Or they may find out how persistence, humor, and caring help more than one might think. Health professionals may find a patient's and families' inner thoughts helpful when considering how best to treat the next Guillain-Barré Syndrome patient they encounter. We sincerely hope so.

"The buildings do not matter much.
Meaning flows from the caregivers."

Erie Chapman
Author *Radical Loving Care*

Chapter One

Onset

Slowly my eyelids blinked open, but only slightly, as I struggled to see the foot of the bed in the grey light of early morning.

Focusing all my effort, I opened my eyes a little wider, taking in the lightweight blanket draped over my body like a white sea stretching from my chin to where it fell off into nothingness. Throughout the night, I had never moved.

The machines beside my bed clicked and whirred while I struggled to pull thoughts together, a task more difficult than keeping my eyes open. Gently the lids closed again, putting me back into my own private world where I could rehearse the sequence of events that had brought me to this place.

Today, I reminded myself, I had been away from my work at the public relations firm for eight days, and it was ten days since the pain first appeared. With no calendar in the room and no clock, I fought feelings of disassociation and struggled to remember that this was Saturday, Day 10.

As I came more fully awake, my thoughts jumped to my clients. Missing a week of work, I knew, would throw every project out of kilter. But on this tenth day I still had hopes of a fast recovery and I wondered how soon I'd be able to call the office for an update.

In retrospect, these thoughts that began each morning when I woke up were unrealistic. I was tied to a ventilator, tubes running in and out of me, monitors beeping, lights flashing all in an effort to keep me alive. Evidently my thoughts were not governed by rationality but by a deep need to keep myself connected to a life that was rapidly receding.

My mind snapped back to the sequence. Day 1 was a week ago Thursday when twinges of pain needled my lower back and behind both knees. That night my husband, Stu, and I had tickets to the Ohio State - Penn State basketball game, a favorite rivalry for us.

Hand in hand Stu and I walked toward the arena in a blustery February wind, falling in with hundreds of fans on the plaza in front of the new red brick basketball arena, glowing with inside light. We pushed our way through knots of people waiting for friends and arm waving entrepreneurs selling the few remaining tickets. It was close to a sellout.

For an hour and a half, we cheered along with a packed house of screaming fans as the score seesawed back and forth. And before we realized it, the final buzzer sounded. Stu remarked about the intensity of the game and the eventual Ohio State victory as we walked through the rising snowstorm that had blown in during the game.

As we walked away from the arena, the pristine snow, sparkling lights, and peaceful quiet seemed right for making snow angels on the sloping hill where the asphalt met the grass. I pulled at his hand,

"Come on, let's make snow angels!"

"Beat you to it," Stu said as he raced to the hillside. I tried to keep up, but he got there first.

Stu revels in the smallest pleasures, never inflated with the importance of his professional career and his many significant accomplishments. He is always ready to enjoy the "now" especially in private moments, unobserved.

We flopped down on the hill. Flap, flap the arms: angel wings. Legs out and back: flowing angel skirts. Amidst giggles and guffaws, Stu pulled me up. Fifty-three years old and still having fun. That nagging pain in my knees and back would probably be gone tomorrow. Why mention it now?

On Day 2, a half day of work was done before a persistent, dull pain in my bones sent me home with thoughts of flu and a weekend in bed. The progress report for our newest client, a $4.1 billion, multi-hospital healthcare merger shaping up on the east coast, was going to have to wait.

Having won the health system contract in early January, my boss, Sandy, and I had been on the run ever since, traveling from Maine to Miami, acquainting ourselves with the players and the issues while we worked on a comprehensive public relations strategy. The stress was more than I had ever experienced before in a long and challenging career.

Early in the morning I felt fine. Yesterday's pain had evaporated overnight – those great recuperative powers I attributed to my genes and regular exercise.

The pace of the business day exerted itself and I slid into the comfort of action, decision-making, and planning.

As the morning hours ticked away, though, I had more trouble focusing on the computer screen and the myriad documents fanned out on the desk. My thoughts kept moving from the written page to the growing pain. It had spread from the lower back and my knees to a generalized pain almost everywhere. It was weighing me down.

Shortly after lunch I alerted the staff, promised renewed diligence on Monday, and prepared to head home. Now certain this nagging pain was the flu, I stuffed the most urgent work into my briefcase, dragged myself to the parking lot two blocks from the office, slumped into my car with help from the Ethiopian parking attendant and edged the car into downtown traffic.

As I drove north, the pain increased noticeably. I thought about a lost weekend in bed, my client work falling even farther behind.

Days 3 and 4 passed in a blur of growing pain, restless sleep, and little food. Piles of paper and notebooks slid off the cream-colored comforter onto the floor. I looked at the mauve fleur de lis on the comforter and thought how pretty they were, a multitude of them cascading over the edge of the bed. I couldn't even think about what was in those papers. The pain was all-consuming, leaving no room in my head for thinking or planning.

Later when Stu came in from work, I heard him quietly open the bedroom door,

"Why are you in bed?"

"I think it's the flu. I ache all over."

"Can I get you anything? A little dinner? Water?"

"No thanks, I'm not hungry."

Neither of us got sick often but through thirty-two years of marriage we had learned to leave each other alone to cope with colds and flu, checking only periodically to provide consolation and offers of liquids, food, or medication. So, Stu nodded his understanding and shut the door while I began my frightening journey alone.

The pain throbbed deeper in every bone and grew more intense. Nothing touched the pain, except water as hot as I could stand flowing out of the shower head, down my back and over the backs of my knees. When I needed relief, I leaned my head against the cool green-grey tile wall letting hot water flow over me for fifteen or twenty minutes. Then a couple of Codeine left over from long ago dental surgery and back into bed.

By Sunday night I couldn't stand the pain any longer. The next time Stu stuck his head into the bedroom I said,

"I really need to go to an emergency room. This pain is unbearable."

"Okay, I'll heat up the car," he offered, concern creasing his brow and showing in his eyes.

I pulled on some loose-fitting clothes and shuffled out to the car. When Stu shut the car door, I lolled to the right like a rag doll with no will to hold myself upright, my eyes closed. I couldn't muster the energy to talk during the forty-minute drive.

The Emergency Department was crowded. Because February is flu season, I suspected that's why so many people were there. But by this time, I was pretty convinced I didn't have the flu. I never had flu without a fever. I never had pain that grew and grew without relenting. I never had the aches and pains of flu that couldn't be controlled with over-the-counter medication.

When the triage nurse finished jotting down my symptoms, my eyes swung toward Stu at the insurance desk. I hoped he would be finished soon as I was having trouble sitting up. Occasionally I slumped to one side, then struggled to push my weight back up to vertical. I no longer had the strength or the will to do it. I felt like I had no bones to give form to my muscles.

When Stu returned, he put his arms around me and gently helped me into a sitting position while he whispered, "Everything is going to be alright." There we sat holding hands, until my turn finally came. Stu supported me as I shuffled down the corridor into the curtain-shrouded cubicle. My legs weren't working very well.

A first-year resident took a brief medical history: pain everywhere and weakness in the legs. Mostly I told him what I didn't have: no fever, no vomiting, and no diarrhea. A nurse took my vital signs. They were close to normal. As usual at a university medical center, a staff physician completed the exam. Blood was drawn for laboratory tests and as we waited for the results, I was given fluids and a snack.

When it came to the question of pain, I was stumped. How do you explain to someone "how much" pain you are in? Using their scale of one to ten, I gave my pain a nine thinking there are probably other forms of pain worse than what I was experiencing even though I couldn't imagine what those were. I was going to find out over the next several months that evaluating pain is subjective and imprecise.

As we waited for a diagnosis, I tried to explain that I was barely able to walk without Stu holding me up. This information was jotted down but didn't seem to make much of an impression. I gave up trying to explain how unusual Stu and I thought this was. I couldn't think beyond the pain and I couldn't explain any better than I had that this was no ordinary flu.

"You have the flu. Take this pain medication and remember to drink lots of liquids," the doctor said as he handed me a prescription.

What we didn't know then was what my medical record revealed when I reviewed it years later. In checking the cranial nerves, which were reported "intact," it was also reported that "deep tendon reflexes are poorly elicited in the patient's lower extremities." This astute observation was not incorporated properly into the diagnosis and wouldn't be fully meaningful until the following day, but it did correlate with the weakness I felt in my legs.

We trudged back to the car and as Stu drove to the closest pharmacy, I felt utter despair. "Here it is," Stu said as he handed the small bag of medicine to me.

The car roared to life with the turn of the ignition and we both stared into the darkness on our way home, not saying a thing. I sensed that Stu knew as well as I did this probably wasn't the flu.

Back home, Stu sat me gently on the side of the bed where I pulled off my sweat clothes lethargically, leaving them in a heap next to the bedside table. He helped pull a comfortable flannel nightgown over my head, planted a gentle kiss on my forehead and, as he squeezed my shoulder, I said, "Why don't you sleep upstairs. I'm so restless, I'll probably keep you awake."

Moonlight flooded through the triple window that looked out to a wooded ravine and swept the opposite wall, lighting this sanctuary Stu and I loved so much. We liked to sit on the small deck outside and watch herds of deer traveling up the valley. Or spot owls soaring through the towering trees. I tried to conjure the good feelings of those times, but the pain would not let me.

I flopped from one side to the other, sat up and looked out the window. Rolled over again and went into the bathroom to take a hot shower. Obviously whatever medication they had given me in the ED wasn't strong enough to deal with this pain. I took the last two Codeine in the bottle and fell into a fitful sleep.

On Monday morning Day 5, awakened by throbbing pain, I swung my legs out of bed and pushed with my hands to launch myself toward the bathroom. As the green-carpeted floor rushed up to meet me, I realized my legs weren't working. The push with my hands sent my upper body forward while my feet hit the floor and my knees buckled, crumpling me into a pile beside the bed.

I felt no fear, just puzzlement. Had I tripped on the comforter? Or was one of my legs asleep? As I tried to collect myself and push up to a standing position, my mind could see what it wanted my body to do, but my legs wouldn't fold up under me like I wanted them to.

Balanced on my right hip, my useless legs stretched out to the side, I flipped onto my stomach, pushed up with both arms and "walked" my body forward inch by inch. In frustration, I shouted for help. My cries summoned our two, boisterous dogs.

Immediately sensing trouble, they circled around me sniffing out the problem. Smokey, the larger of the two, licked my face. I smiled a little as his large pink tongue swept over my cheek. A combination Irish wolfhound and black Labrador retriever, he towered over me cocking his head from one side to the other, raising an eyebrow as if to ask, "What's the matter with you?"

Max was much smaller, older, and calmer than Smokey. He circled me several times, then backed away as though he knew something bad was happening.

Confused and starting to panic, I extended my arms, gripped the forest green carpet and pulled, dragging my useless legs behind me like an inchworm with a broken back third. I advanced slowly until I crossed the threshold into the hallway. The dogs kept their distance, circling and sniffing.

My mind raced with questions and a refusal to accept what was happening. Why wouldn't my ankles or knees bend? Why couldn't I stand up? What was happening to me?

Stu, in plaid pajama bottoms and a blue T-shirt, bounded into our bedroom where he found me crying softly and saying, "I can't move my legs." Stu looked terrified as I told him the horrid news.

Brushing the dogs aside, he kneeled beside me, considering how to lift me from the floor. Stu leveraged his arms under my shoulders, then pulled me upward as he staggered to a standing position. We clung to each other, desperately wondering what was happening.

"Why can't I walk, Stu?" I whispered.

"I don't know."

My heart sank and tears rolled down my cheeks as I realized my legs were paralyzed.

Chapter Two

Diagnosis

I 've been in the healthcare world, albeit as a hospital CEO and not a clinician, since my graduate work at the University of Chicago. I had never heard of anything like this. There must be some simple answer, I told myself, but didn't speculate with Carole. Frightening thoughts rolled around in my head as we drove toward the hospital.

I pulled in under the covered entry to the Emergency Department and grabbed a wheelchair from just inside the automatic doors.

Carole leaned over my left shoulder as I lifted her out of the car and lowered her into the wheelchair. She grimaced and winked in one movement and that told me a lot without saying a word. She was petrified but composed. Like me, she had processed the situation a hundred times during our drive to OSU and had not come up with a logical answer.

As I searched for a parking spot, I thought about the class of graduate students in the School of Public Health I had planned to teach later this morning. I'd have to call my friend and colleague, Steve L, to let him know I wouldn't be there.

As I ran toward the Emergency entrance from a distant parking place, I was startled when I saw Carole huddled in the wheelchair, the orange glow of inside light surrounding her, a stark contrast to the inky blackness outside. She looked so vulnerable and my heart ached for her.

Marshalling thirty years of hospital management experience, I knew I could hurry the check-in along given Carole's dire symptoms. Besides, we had been here the night before so her history and diagnosis were in their computer system already.

My experience as the CEO of the OSU-affiliated Columbus Children's Hospital made me comfortable negotiating what otherwise could have been a very intimidating environment. While I did not realize it at the time, that *grounding would prove to be invaluable as Carole actually, and I, virtually, would be living within these walls for the next five months.*

The first six hours in the Emergency Department were agonizing for both of us. My condition was acute and doctors began their assessment immediately, but there was no cubicle available when we arrived, so I was placed on a gurney, covered with a white sheet, and left in the hallway to stare up at the even rows of little black dots in the tiled ceiling.

People hurried by on their way to green-draped cubicles. Nurses carried specimens away from patients and sent them to the laboratory. Doctors moved from patient to patient, questioning, assessing, or explaining a diagnosis.

"Will you be OK for a while? I want to go talk to the doctors."

"Yes, I don't plan on going anywhere," I joked feebly.

"I'll be back soon," Stu said in an effort to comfort me, but I could see the anxiety in his eyes.

The wait seemed endless. I counted the dots on the ceiling for the sixth time and wondered why no one was talking to me. I took both arms out from under the sheet and clasped my hands over my stomach. More counting. More watching. It seemed like hours since our arrival and Stu hadn't stopped by in a long time.

Finally, Stu returned to my gurney, grabbed my hand and told me a cubicle was available now. As an attendant rolled the gurney through the wide pathway past the bustling nurses' station, Stu hurried alongside describing the discussions physicians were having about my case. He said progress was being made toward making a diagnosis, but didn't elaborate.

Once two attendants transferred me to a bed, the questioning began. One doctor after another asked about my recent illness, any other symptoms I might have noticed, how I was feeling now. My reflexes were checked. There were none in my feet or legs below the knee, but all others were normal. All I could tell them was,

"In some ways this feels like the flu but the only symptom I have is pain and, now, paralysis. I was perfectly healthy last Thursday."

Time is a marvelous commodity. When you are experiencing a pleasant event, time rushes by like rapids through a canyon. Despite your efforts to slow the current and enjoy the moment, it's over too soon and you remember the exhilaration more than the event itself. As you plow your way through a frightening journey with an unknown outcome, time slows to a methodical drip. Yet, as you look back to recall it, you only remember a blur. The painful emotions attached to the trial of waiting may stay with you forever. That's how I felt on Monday morning.

A parade of interns, residents, and medical students flowed in and out of Carole's curtained cubicle playing out a diagnostic process I knew well. Teaching hospitals involve medical students in the evaluation of patients' conditions and diagnoses of their illnesses.

The known facts about the patient are given to the medical students and junior residents and each is challenged to consider alternative causes and future courses of action. Were more tests required? More information from the patient? Think hard! What are we dealing with?

The attending physicians challenge everyone in the room. In the first hour or so Carole was questioned relentlessly and repetitively.

Then residents with different medical specialties arrived in her cubicle. Emergency Department residents got first crack at Carole's case followed by an internal medicine resident. Soon neurology residents appeared in response to a call for more expertise.

I knew that behind this veil of young physicians and students in short white coats was a knowledgeable faculty supervising a process both fascinating and productive. Students' inquisitive minds searched for answers and at the same time challenged their professors with probing questions keeping them on top of their game. This team of experts brought an incredible body of knowledge and expertise to bear on Carole's case.

Following the preliminary diagnosis which I interpreted as, "Carole, you have something far more serious than the flu," we were relocated to a room off the main emergency center which gave us privacy as well as anxious concern. Was this because an alert clerk had picked up from the insurance information that I had been the CEO of the cross-town children's hospital? Or, was Carole's situation grave enough that they wanted to give her some privacy for what she was about to hear?

Now they were processing blood and urine tests through the laboratory. A stat label would take Carole's lab samples to the front of the line but in a place the size of OSU, there would be hundreds of tests to process. The granules of sand in the imaginary hourglass dropped one by one into the lower chamber.

We talked about our kids and what they might be doing. Katie, our youngest, would be trudging through Pennsylvania's winter snow to one of her senior classes at Allegheny College. I glanced at my watch. It must have stopped.

Glen, our middle child, would be sleeping after closing down the restaurant he managed in German Village, just south of the city. Would he be seeing that cute little blond server he worked with later in the day?

I wondered how many things could slow down the processing of a stat lab test. What if they had misplaced the vials? I glanced down: the hands on my watch seemed to be moving again.

Our first born, Eric, was working in Washington, D.C. while completing his Master of Fine Arts (MFA) degree at Columbia University. Soon he would storm Hollywood, scripts in hand with hopes of getting a movie deal.

After a soft knock, the senior resident opened the door. He explained that one more test would be necessary to confirm a diagnosis. He needed to draw some spinal fluid from Carole's back. After the necessary disclaimers mixed with the reassurance he had done "hundreds of spinal taps," Carole signed the authorization form then rolled onto her side and curled into a ball exposing the spaces between her vertebrae.

The procedure took only a few minutes. As she settled back on the pillow, I saw tears in Carole's eyes. I knew they were not from any pain the needle might have caused, but from fear of the unknown. This morning we'd been dropped together into a dark hole and we weren't sure yet how to get out. We looked at each other and knew we were sharing the same fear. I squeezed her hand and said, "We'll get through this together."

While we waited for the test results, I cornered the senior resident and quizzed him about what we might be dealing with. He was very forthright and explained,

> *"There are several possibilities: Polio, Hodgkin's Disease, Muscular Dystrophy, Multiple Sclerosis, or Guillain-Barré Syndrome."*

> *"I've never heard of Guillain-Barré, but I don't like the sound of any of the other alternatives."*

> *"We've already eliminated several diseases and I'm putting my money on Guillain-Barré Syndrome. I'll know more when I see the results of the spinal tap."*

Finally, the exam room door handle turned and the resident entered with a professional look on his face. In that frozen moment, I tried to read his mind. Good news? Terrible news? He rolled the metal stool up to the bed and sat so his face was level with Carole's.

> *"Carole, the bottom line is you have what is known as Guillain-Barré Syndrome."*

The young, well-mannered resident was impressive. He was calm and direct but seemed to understand the message he was delivering was a bombshell. He looked at and talked directly to Carole. I saw and heard every word like a slow-motion film, portions of the explanation etched on my brain like a tattoo.

Guillain-Barré Syndrome (GBS) is a disease of unknown origin and is very rare. Fourteen people per million contract it each year. The resident explained that its onset seems to be correlated to receiving a flu vaccination or having an infection, several weeks before the onset of the disease itself. It might also be caused by camphlobacter jejuni, a bacterium found in well water and in some raw chicken. Whatever the instigator, the body's immune system attacks the body itself, as if it were a foreign intruder. The attack is concentrated on the myelin sheath that covers all the nerves in the body.*

The myelin sheath protects the nerves as they do their job of conveying electrical impulses from the brain to all the muscles in the body. This intricate process is abruptly interrupted by the onset of Guillain-Barré Syndrome as the myelin sheath dissolves. The young resident went on,

> *"Typically, but not always, GBS launches its attack in the feet and gradually works its way up the body, then slowly reverses as the myelin sheath regenerates."*

> *"How far will it move up my body?" Carole asked.*

> *"The plateau is usually at the knees or waist but it can go higher and in extremely rare cases engage the entire body." I asked,*

> *"Is there a cure?"*

> *"No," the resident responded, "there really is no cure. We can only treat the symptoms, control the pain, and let the disease run its course."*

> *"At some point, the damage levels off and then slowly begins to reverse as the myelin sheath grows back. Theoretically, the repair will be complete and the body will eventually return to its normal condition."*

My mind caught on certain words and phrases: **Theoretically**, *the repair will be complete......it can go* **higher......**consume the **entire body......no cure......**treat the **symptoms......it takes time......how far it travels** and how **much damage is done.***

---

* Medical Appendix. Deterioration of the Myelin Sheath.

I stared at the ceiling, the young resident, and then at Carole. She looked scared to death.

Dr. M, the neurologist in charge of my case, explained Guillain-Barré Syndrome * and what to expect next. It was a description similar to what the resident had told us, but neither explanation prepared us for what was to come. One thing he said did stick in my head, "Don't worry, 80 percent of patients get 100 percent recovery."

As Dr. M continued, I recalled a story shared six months earlier by a friend. Late one night her daughter had phoned from Denver. She was lying on the bathroom floor unable to move her legs and didn't know what was wrong. Her mother told her to hang up and call an ambulance. The daughter was rushed to the hospital where the paralysis proceeded to her waist, halted and then, over time, retreated. By the time her mother told me the story, her daughter was fully recovered from her encounter with Guillain-Barré Syndrome.

As Dr. M finished his explanation, I hoped my experience would be similar to my friend's daughter. The paralysis might progress to my waist but would soon reverse itself and I'd be headed home.

---

* Medical Appendix. What is Guillain-Barre Syndrome?

Chapter Three

On the Move

Days 5, 6, and 7 dragged by. Early each morning my neurologist, with accompanying medical students and residents, came to assess the progress of the paralysis. They asked questions and discussed my condition, but told me nothing I couldn't see for myself.

Monday evening, after admission, I could easily move my thighs and shift my hips from side to side. But by late Wednesday I could no longer move my hips at all. My trunk and arms moved normally, but I admitted to Stu late on Wednesday that my fingers were tingling. My grip was growing weaker. And with this admission, my heart sank. The paralysis was still on the move.

On Thursday, Day 8, I signed authorization for a trach to be inserted into my throat as a precaution against the paralysis moving up to my diaphragm thus compromising my ability to breathe on my own.* He explained the need briefly and logically, leaning over the bed and looking directly at me. Dressed in a long white physician's coat, he had a distinguished look about him. I noticed his grey hair was combed neatly as the doctor explained the reasons for inserting the trach now. He consoled me by saying,

"It probably won't be necessary to attach you to a ventilator. We're just doing this as a precaution."

"Okay," I mumbled, realizing this meant the paralysis was still moving up my body and a small voice in my head said, "If this happens, you won't be able to talk."

Stu hung in the background letting me work with the physician on this issue. I wondered and I worried as they wheeled my bed to surgery, "Would it have been better to wait to see if the paralysis stopped where it was?"

---

* Medical Appendix. Nerves that Control the Diaphragm.

Thankfully it wasn't long before anesthesia eased me into a black pit of nothingness. When I woke, I was back in my room, a trach sticking out of my throat. I could still breathe and talk on my own.

On his next visit to my room, Dr. M explained how GBS (in years past known as Landry's Ascending Paralysis)* would continue to move upward and then, for unknown reasons, reverse course and retreat. He repeated his mantra that "80 percent of Guillain-Barré patients get 100 percent recovery," a prognosis that both encouraged and terrified me. Of course, since first hearing this statistic, I hoped to be in the 80 percent and yet was never told what, exactly, happened to the other 20 percent. He also reminded me that the progression could stop at any time and they were hopeful I would not have to be placed on the ventilator.

Dr. M continued to test my reflexes each day. By now it was a certainty there would be no response below my waist. Although my grip was growing weaker, I was still able to raise my arms, grasp his fingers, and squeeze.

While I clung to what was left of movement in my upper body, I was terrified of what else I might lose. What if I lost the use of my hands? Would I be placed on the ventilator? How, I wondered, do you ever get off a ventilator? If Stu was asking the neurologist these questions, he never volunteered what he was learning.

On Day 9, it was obvious the trach decision had been the right one. The doctors told me it was time to attach the ventilator to the tube in my neck. Doubt, concern, fear, and anger pin-balled around in my head.

"No, this isn't possible! I can still breathe on my own."

The pulmonologist assured me quietly,

"We must attach you to the ventilator now, Carole. The paralysis is still moving upward and will soon compromise your breathing. Waiting for the moment when you actually stop breathing would be dangerous."

I closed my eyes and fought back tears as I listened to the quiet "whoosh, whoosh" of the machine at the side of my bed. A nurse had reclined the bed before attaching the ventilator to my trach with a long, flexible hose. I looked up at the ceiling with those long rows of parallel dots and resigned myself to reality: I could no longer breathe on my own or speak for myself. Tears dropped quietly from my eyes, splashing into my ears while others soaked the pillow on both sides of my head.

---

* Medical Appendix. A Brief History of GBS.

There hadn't been time to formulate my last few words before going silent. Although, until now, I had kept a brave front for Stu, my confidence slipped when they attached me to that machine. I looked beyond the nurse and realized then that I wouldn't be able to interact with the physicians, ask my own questions, or explore what was happening to me. I couldn't tell Stu what was troubling me or reassure him that I could fight this. I wanted to ask him to hold me and comfort me now that I had lost all hope. But instead I stared at him glumly and thought how dejected and sad he looked, a mirror of my own feelings.

As I listened in silence that evening, Stu wondered aloud why my fingers had begun to tingle the day before. Wouldn't the paralysis be expected to move up from the feet and out from the spine? Wouldn't it move from the shoulders down the arms and into the hands? Instead it seemed to be going in reverse now. Stu described GBS as "a sadistic bastard" who invented ways to torment its victims.

With the paralysis moving more quickly now, Dr. M ordered a course of Intravenous Immunoglobulin (IVIg), one of two treatments used on GBS patients. Immunoglobulin is made from antibodies filtered out of donated human blood and suspended in a sterile solution. Because GBS is an autoimmune disease in which antibodies attack the peripheral nerves, it is hoped administration of IVIg will slow or reverse this process.*

The paralysis seemed to move more quickly once I was on the ventilator. It rushed from my hands upward through my arms as morning dwindled away. The nurse lowered the bed to the fully reclined position as I started losing feeling in my face. All I felt was total dread.

That afternoon a friend stuck her head into the room to say "hello." She gave me a rag doll angel. It was white with curly brown hair, large fabric wings, and a body of fabric streamers cut in a profusion of strips. The round face was painted with rosy pink cheeks and a round "O" for a mouth. It was a lovely gift delivered at just the right time for in a few minutes my room was in chaos.

My friend was gently pushed out of the room while doctors and nurses talking in clipped directives collected my things, piling the bed with tubing and monitors, responding to an order for immediate evacuation to the ICU where I could be more closely monitored. I heard whispers of "worst possible scenario." My heart beat rapidly.

---

* Medical Appendix: IVIg and Plasmapheresis.

Like a heart-wrenching TV episode where a roomful of doctors and nurses strive heroically to save the patient, I felt like I was in a staged drama. But this was real and I was the patient.

No one told me what was happening, but four people rapidly lifted me onto a gurney. The ventilator whooshed beside me and the little white angel lay on my inert body among a jumble of tubes and bags where she rode with me to the ICU. I twisted my head from side to side looking for Stu. But he wasn't there. My mind raced even faster than my heart.

The past week had been a nightmare, but Saturday, I will never forget. The sadistic GBS phantom had stolen everything but Carole's eyes. I had been warned at the nursing station before going into her room that the paralysis had progressed into her face, but nothing could have prepared me for what remained of the attractive girl I had fallen in love with as a senior in high school; the young lady I had married after we both graduated from college; the woman I had shared every dream, ambition, and problem with for the last twenty-five years; the one who brought our three children into the world and the playful friend I'd made snow angels with just a week before.

She was flat on her back looking up at the ceiling, her face muscles sagging. The only other times I had witnessed such a complete lack of expression was at open casket funerals. It hit me like a truck out of total darkness. The only glimpse I had of my Carole was through her dark brown eyes.

There were tears in both our eyes. She couldn't speak but there was a huge message coming out of those eyes. As I stood looking at her, she blinked! That blink seemed like a relatively small thing at the time but turned out to be a tremendous advantage in the weeks that followed. What was she thinking behind the deep black pools of those eyes?

"Help! All I can do is blink! I can't move anything! I can't talk. I'm trapped in my own body. Stu, please help me."

Later that morning the chief resident and I discussed the need to tape Carole's eyes shut to protect the remaining moisture in her eyes. I pleaded, argued, and cajoled.

"She can still blink on her own. Taping her eyes closed will shut the only door she has to reality," I argued.

"It would be best to tape her eyes shut," the resident urged.

"Can't you use eye drops or moist clothes to keep her eyes lubricated?"

Finally, the resident agreed to delay his decision and assess it day-by-day. In the meantime, eye drops would be administered.

"Carole," I said, "they're going to give you eye drops." I almost choked on the words as I saw so much fear in her eyes. "I love you so much. Just remember, it's important to keep blinking."

The last muscles in her body held on. If her eyelids had failed, the doctors would have had no alternative but to tape her eyes shut, extinguishing all light in her already very dark world.

Our prayers were separate and silent. Carole had no choice and I needed to let my thoughts form themselves into prayers. Our religious beliefs are basic and not particularly fervent. We prayed to a God of whose form we were not sure. We liked to believe He intercedes and helps people in need. I'm not sure this is the case, but if He does, this would be a great time for Him to step in. "Please, God, help her through this. Help me to help her."

Just as these words passed through my mind, a nurse informed me Carole would be moved to the Intensive Care Unit (ICU) on the tenth floor where she could be monitored twenty-four hours a day.

Day 10.

Hope struggled to keep a place in my mind, but each day I found it harder to remember which day it was, harder to reconstruct even one client's account, impossible to develop next steps as I had always done in the past. On Day 10 I admitted to myself that the fast-paced, multi-tasking person I used to be was lost. I could only concentrate on the Carole that lived inside my head – hoping, wishing, and praying she could recover. A GBS Foundation pamphlet presents my case starkly: "A rare patient may experience total paralysis without ability to move a finger, shrug a shoulder, or blink an eye. Such patients may be effectively 'locked in' or unable to communicate." Indeed. That was me.

While Carole slept. I glanced up at the bag of liquid hanging on a pole beside the bed, draining through a tube into her nose and down into her stomach. The liquid was blue, a trace of the surreal keeping Carole alive. I found out from the head nurse that it is blue because nothing in the body is naturally blue, so if the liquid came out of Carole's trach, they would know it had gone down the wrong tube. Incredible to me.

Regrettably, certain images cannot be erased from the memory. Carole lay utterly still, her eyes closed. There was no smiling, or wincing, or frowning. Her face was as blank as a death mask.

❋ ❋ ❋

Stu knew my mind was alive, searching for answers, wondering what was happening, hoping for explanations, and longing for relief from the constant pain. Most remarkable was his determination to bring the "real" me to the fore. I watched and listened as Stu explained who I was, what I used to look like, and that I was still here, looking out, wanting desperately to talk, and wanting even more desperately to participate in getting well.

Opportunities to maintain the real me came every day in large and small ways. Not taping my eyes shut was the first big triumph. I could see Stu and tell him with my eyes whether things were going well or not. Seeing those who were discussing my condition made it more real for me and I felt a little bit of participation in every deliberation.

Months after leaving the hospital, I visited a woman with GBS and her supportive family who were going through the agony of deciding how to direct her care. Her doctors recommended she be sedated indefinitely until her condition improved. I was horrified at this recommendation, but this family chose to follow their doctors' advice. When I was in her position, though I couldn't move or talk, I was grateful to have my eyes and my active mind. I was so glad never to have been sedated into oblivion.

To my relief, by Sunday morning when I walked into her room, Carole had a little bit of expression on her face. It was slight, perhaps insignificant to anyone else, but I could see Carole, not just in her eyes, but also in her face. There was a bit of attitude. There was life.

To explain to Carole on Sunday, how much better she looked than she had the day before just didn't seem to fit into a morning greeting. She was still 99 percent paralyzed. I didn't think about it at the time, but GBS had probably reached its peak and begun its long, slow process of repair to the myelin sheath.

That afternoon as Carole awoke from a nap, she blinked, moved her head slowly from side to side, then looked straight ahead gazing into the distance. Her ability to communicate had been reduced to her heart rate, blood pressure, and her eyes.

I sensed her utter frustration. Gently, I pulled her chin around until she could look into my eyes. Love, relaxation, confidence, concern, questions, fear... they were all there, in the eyes. How could I help them get out?

To make healthy Carole a reality to medical personnel, Stu tacked a recent photo of me to the wall above the bed. Then, he started making frequent references to my preferences, my ideas, my hopes. He stated them as if he were channeling my very thoughts.

And he set a small CD player on the bedside table, playing music whenever he was there and never failed to insert a CD before he left. But many times, when he returned for a visit, no music was playing. So, he posted a sign: *When you leave this room, please insert a new CD.* Brilliant! Now I had a variety of music day and night.

This mental stimulation was helpful in the lonely evenings when I stared up at the ceiling or out the glass door toward the nurses' station buzzing with activity but far removed from my own experience.

For long stretches when I lay listening to classical music, I thought of others in comparable circumstances. I wondered about prisoners of war and people who suffered from ALS. How did they keep their minds active? Some, I had read, relived, mentally, their entire lives. Others played chess-in-the-head or planned their futures post-imprisonment. I tried each of these but had no success. My mind wandered from each task I set for myself, seeking relief from the pain, turning away from contemplation and resting in the music.

Not being able to communicate her thoughts to medical personnel was a problem in so many ways. Because Carole couldn't move or talk, some caregivers simply ignored her. She wasn't responsive, so why try to communicate? Others tried to soothe her by patting or rubbing her arm while talking to her. The problem was, a pat or rub on the arm was like drilling a tooth without Novocain. Or stroking a burn patient to the point of rubbing off the skin. Because Carole could not talk, scream, or cry out, caregivers had no idea of their transgressions. Eventually I explained the problem to the staff, but I don't believe they, or I, ever realized the nightmare Carole was experiencing.

Chapter Four

Pain in the ICU

The pain was unbearable and of three kinds. Every bone throbbed like an infected tooth. Muscular and ligament pain was akin to a badly sprained ankle. And my skin was sensitive to the lightest touch, much worse than any sunburn I'd ever experienced. I couldn't tolerate the slightest touch of my skin.

While physicians certainly understand that severe pain can be a factor in about a quarter of GBS cases,[*] they don't have any indication of its severity – especially if the patient is rendered speechless. Just as it was during my visit to the Emergency Department, no one seemed to believe I could be in this much pain. In the first few days in the hospital, when I still had a voice, I failed in every attempt to explain how much pain I was in. Painkillers were administered, but they gave relief for only a short time or not at all.

Once I lay speechless in the ICU, I could no longer describe the pain coursing through my body. Perhaps responding to Stu's constant references to the pain I described before falling silent, the doctors kept this aspect of GBS in mind.

After trying several medications without relieving the agony, the attending physician ordered a morphine drip. Finally, this worked to ease the pain, but now I was enslaved to a cycle: total freedom from pain when morphine was added to the saline solution bag, followed by diminished relief as the drug ran out. As the pain increased, my internal anxiety mounted. I listened for the subtle squeaking of shoes on the floor, hoping someone was coming to give me the next dose.

One issue the ICU staff faced is the rarity of Guillain-Barré Syndrome. Many cases are so mild, they require no hospitalization, so while the ICU staff

---

[*] Medical Appendix. Pain in GBS.

was very skilled and professional, the last GBS patient requiring ICU care may have been admitted years ago.

As a hospital CEO, I knew the challenge facing the head nurse. With three shifts a day, seven days a week and backup sufficient to cover vacations, holidays, and sick days, she had to consider how to bring more than fifty professional staff plus aides and housekeeping personnel up to speed on the unique issues Carole was facing.

For the first few days, Stu did not tell many people what was happening to me. He hoped, as I did, that the debilitation of Guillain-Barré Syndrome would reverse quickly and I would soon go home. But by Friday we knew this was not going to happen and he began contacting family and friends.

One morning the second week of this ordeal, our oldest son Eric appeared beside my bed. Subdued but smiling, he talked easily about what he could do to help. That this meant I was desperately ill didn't even cross my mind, but it probably should have.

It was both encouraging and frightening to watch Eric's reaction as he stared down at me. His physique is like Stu's, both about 5' 10" tall with a medium build. His brown hair was cut close and his generous, warm smile reminded me of Stu's. I looked out with a happiness I could not show and he stared at me with a startled fear he tried to hide behind that wonderful smile.

I expected Eric to check out my condition, offer support, and get back to his own life in Washington, D.C., but he chose that day to move home to support us through our horrendous challenges.

Our other two children, second son Glen and daughter Katie, were not as available to help as Eric was. Glen lived in town but worked a grueling restaurant schedule and Katie was almost two hundred miles away finishing her last semester of college. But I should have known they'd both be on their way to see us as soon as they heard the news.

The elevator's stilted computer voice announced its arrival at the tenth floor whenever Glen came to visit. He always turned left heading for the visitors' lounge intentionally avoiding the metal-clad doors that swing into the ICU corridor. He sat in the lounge and stared straight ahead. Stu asked Glen,

"Don't you want to come in and see Mom?"

"No. I'll just sit here. Please tell her I love her and thinking about her."

"Come on, Glen. She wants to see you.

"I can't do it. I'll be here for a while."

Glen might have wondered if I was going to make it. Or maybe he was just numb not knowing what to do or how to act. For days Stu encouraged Glen to enter my room,

"Come in and see Mom today, Glen."

"Does she have tubes in?"

"Yes, but she's going to recover, Glen, and I know she wants to see you."

"I don't know what to say."

"It will help Mom to see you."

I'll never forget the first day Glen edged into my room. He came in quietly so I didn't see him at first. He was standing behind Stu out of my line of sight. Then Stu said quietly, "Glen's here." I rolled my eyes to the left as Glen took two steps closer to the bed. He seemed stiff, unnatural, and awkward. He didn't say a word. Eric filled the void, trying to help Glen feel more comfortable. Finally, Glen took a step closer to the bed. He leaned over and said

"Mom, your lips are chapped."

He reached over and gently spread mint-flavored Chapstick on my lips. I believe that's the only thing he said that day. And every day after that, Glen always brought Chapstick to the hospital and lovingly fought off my dry lips. It touched me deeply. How different our two sons are. Each had found his own way to reach through the isolation, the pain, paralysis, and drugs to touch my heart. While each method of communication was different, the message of love, concern, and compassion was the same.

Glen didn't know but his gesture was the same one I had used when my father lay dying in Pittsburgh years earlier. When I visited my father during his terminal illness, I think I felt much as Glen did when he came to visit me. As the family waited in the visitors' lounge each anticipating their turn alone with my father, I was fearful. I didn't know what to say or do. When my turn came, I edged up next to his bed. I could see in his eyes that his mind was active, that he wanted to talk. I saw tears pool in the corners of his eyes as he considered the sadness of the end of life and I thought I saw anger at the unfairness of dying too young and without being able to voice his goodbyes. But unlike Eric with me, I never said a word to my father. I reacted much more as Glen had with me. I sat with Dad. I looked into his eyes. I touched the covers that were neatly tucked up to his chin to cover his paralyzed body. I couldn't think of a thing to say.

Years later I hated myself for not understanding that my Dad wanted me to talk to him, to ask questions, to find a way for him to communicate with me. I tried to comfort him just by being there. So, I understood Glen perfectly seventeen years later when he did the same for me. And, like Glen, I swabbed my father's lips with balm to ease the chapping. In my own hospital bed, I came to the realization my father probably understood my thoughts just as I understood Glen's.

Katie was a world away mentally from my worsening condition. I didn't expect she would be able to take time away from her preparation to defend her senior thesis on snow leopards' adaptation to zoo environments. I imagined Stu had not conveyed the seriousness of my situation both to protect her from worry and to bolster his own hope that everything would work out for the best.

But obviously he had, because very soon Katie arrived in Columbus, boyfriend in tow, to bring me her love, consolation, cheer, and hope. I treasured her face near mine trying to talk of relevant things when she knew nothing was as relevant as struggling to live. Those things, though, you don't put into words. Hope lives in family connections and returning to normal and that is the gift Katie gave me.

And I can still see Keith, my son-in-law-to-be, the first time they came to visit, standing ramrod straight against the wall all six foot two of him gazing at someone he had never met, lying immobile and silent. What could he possibly say? Wisely, he didn't try, but I was hoping in the weeks to come he would be a comfort to Katie.

When he turned to leave the room, I saw his eight-inch ponytail protruding from the hole in the back of his baseball cap. I couldn't wait to talk with this young man who had captured Katie's heart!

As I arrived on a frigid February morning at the ICU, a new shift of nurses was coming on duty. I introduced myself to the head nurse and asked,

> *"How's Carole doing?"*

> *"She's doing fine. She's stable and her vital signs are where we would expect them to be."*

What was not said was,

> *"She's a lot better. She's sitting up and asking about you and the kids."*

She was stable and that was it. My heart sank.

I mentally willed myself to enter her glass enclosure and leaned down, my head hovering over her face. Her eyes were closed so I just lightly kissed her forehead. Her eyelids blinked open, then slowly shut. They opened again.

Instantly we made a connection. Her mind was easy to read. "I love you. Can we go home soon?" I answered the first half of her message but ignored the second. "I love you, too."

Because she couldn't talk, I felt the need to fill the void with my own voice. I told her about some of the people who had called and wanted me to pass on their good wishes. As I looked at her face, she was blinking rapidly. So rapidly, I almost called the nurse. After she realized I had noticed her blinks, she rolled her eyes side to side. I bent over her with our faces less than a foot apart. She blinked once. Then she blinked twice. Then three times. She was showing me she could blink out a message.

"Are you trying to tell me something?"

Two blinks, which I took to mean, "YES."

I felt a surge of wonder as I had when astronaut Neil Armstrong communicated from the moon back to earth. We had just communicated back and forth for the first time in eleven days.

From that point, we made progress in our communication challenge. The first stage was asking Carole questions she could answer with two blinks, a Yes, or one blink, a No. That "conversation" lasted about thirty minutes when it became apparent this was still pretty much one-way communication.

Later that day, I mentioned the communication conundrum to Carole's social worker. She left the ICU and returned shortly with an alphabet board, a standard tool used with patients unable to talk.

I slid my finger along the letters waiting for Carole to signal with a blink when I hit the right letter. The first message she sent me, "I-LOVE-YOU." With difficulty, I held back my tears.

The second message started, P-L-E-A-S-E.

"Carole," I pleaded, "Whatever you need, don't start the sentence with please." The message continued, "R-E-A-R."

I needed no more letters for I knew where she was going. "You have an issue with your butt. I'll call the nurse!"

Three hard blinks from Carole and I waited while she started the message again.

R-E-A-R-R-A-N-G-E M-Y L-E-G-S.

I put the pad down and rearranged her legs before pointing out the benefits of using short words like "move" instead of "rearrange."

Every time Stu arrived in my room, he was smiling and positive. He brought new information, greetings from friends, and the promise of visits from family members. I didn't realize until much later the incredible amount of pressure and fear he was feeling. Because so little is known about GBS and cases can vary so widely, he couldn't figure out what might be in store.

Stu seemed to be everywhere at once, talking to doctors and nurses, letting me know their current thinking. He told me a second round of IVIg had been prescribed by Dr. M and would be started soon. This was the second five-day course administered since admission. I wondered why we weren't seeing any improvement if this was a promising therapy.

Eric and Stu organized the days into shifts each spelling the other and, at times, doubling up their visits carrying on enthusiastic three-way conversations with me as their silent partner.

Eric's creative mind went right to work identifying ways to entertain me, to pass the time, and to keep my spirits up. One day he brought in a stack of novels, read all the titles, and asked me to choose the one I'd like to hear. I chose "Mosquito Coast."

As I recall, an aggressive and determined father lead his family into a remote jungle, encountering extraordinary challenges and severe living conditions. As Eric began reading, I transported myself out of my pain and into the elaborate story. This was an excellent vehicle to take me away from myself and so much easier than trying to generate my own thoughts.

Eric had taped a large poster of the American West to the ceiling above my bed. Green grass grew in the foreground and mountains rolled into the distance, a river flowing from the mid-left through the picture to the right front. People and their farm animals traveled through the landscape.

As Eric read "Mosquito Coast," scenes of South America unfolded in my mind as the family found itself isolated and struggling to establish their home. I pictured the lush jungle with trailing vines, colorful flowers and oppressive heat. I closed my eyes and saw the novel's characters playing out their lives. But when I opened my eyes again, the characters moved inexplicably from the jungles of South America to the tranquil countryside in the poster Eric had taped to the ceiling.

There I saw them conducting their lives in unfamiliar territory, not in a South American jungle, but in the American West. My eyes were open. Eric was reading from the chair beside the bed. And I was experiencing the novel in real time on the ceiling of my hospital room. Somehow my mind accepted the anomaly of Mosquito Coast on the ceiling whenever this drug-affected mental motion picture whirred into action.

One day, Eric asked if I wanted him to keep reading this book.

"Pages left?" I blinked

"About 350," was the answer.

"Stop. Too long," so we abandoned Mosquito Coast.

Every day I saw the discarded paperback resting on a stack of all the things Eric had brought into my room to entertain me. It made me sad. He was trying so hard to keep my mind active, but I couldn't concentrate long enough to make most of his efforts worthwhile.

Next, Eric read the evening paper to me. He started by reading a headline with a question mark in his voice. Did I want to hear that article? He read those when I blinked "yes" and skipped the "no's." This was an excellent way to control the length of my exposure to thinking. If I had the interest and stamina, I could listen to an entire article. I liked the ones about city politics, economic development, and international relations. For most others, I blinked, "No."

Eric realized that I needed a way to communicate more specifically than just to blink Yes or No, and more quickly than using the alphabet board. Together he and Stu devised a more useful scheme: a chart with five circles, each containing five or six letters. The person holding the chart pointed to each circle in succession until I blinked. Stopping at that circle, my collaborator then pointed to each letter in the circle until I blinked again, designating the preferred letter.

Remembering Stu's rules about brevity, the first time I used the chart, I blinked, "contact lenses still in!" I had a gnawing feeling that since the onset of GBS, I had not taken my lenses out. Of course, this was untrue as I had come to the hospital right out of bed with no time to put the lenses in.

Physicians peered into my eyes and concluded I was mistaken. While they leaned over me trying to find those lenses in my eyes, I hallucinated a coat hanger dangling next to one doctor's ear with filmy threads hanging off the corner undulating softly. As he assured Stu and Eric there were no contact lenses in my eyes, the dangling coat hanger faded away leaving the filmy threads floating there. I wondered if anyone else could see these things

There were other hallucinations, even more bizarre and in retrospect quite funny. One afternoon I blinked out a complex message to let Stu know he should bring horses to the back of the hospital so we could escape.

Subconsciously I guess morphine helped me find a way to do what I most wanted, to go home.

And some of my best morphine-induced experiences happened when I was alone. The poster on the ceiling was the perfect vehicle. My best trick was to gaze at the poster intently until the colors swirled and the people moved. I could create new animals, multiply the people and make them all move purposefully through the landscape. Greens, browns, and grays dominated the real poster. My morphine poster exploded in reds and yellows against a brilliant blue sky while the mountains grew larger and the river flowed faster. I saw myself there, walking again.

Our communication process improved each time we tried, but it was utterly frustrating for all of us as I struggled to put into very few words the medical travails that plagued me every day. And the procedure was so time-consuming and cumbersome there was no way to have a meaningful or thoughtful conversation about anything other than medical necessities. The rest of what I was thinking and feeling had to stay within myself.

After two weeks, my condition still perilous, I remained in the ICU. I feared being alone and worried about what hospital personnel might do to me when no family member was present, making me glad Stu found ways to provide as much family companionship as possible.

Eric and Stu divided their hospital time into day and evening shifts, and my sister Bonnie, who lived in town, relieved them when she wasn't working.

On Bonnie's work "weekend," Monday and Tuesday, she spent hours in my room, a devoted and cheerful presence who made paper flowers, shared family stories, or sat quietly beside me while I slept.

When her slender 5' 3" frame slid through the glass door, it made me happy to see her cheerful smile light up her large, dark brown eyes. No matter what she thought of my condition, she kept a brave front, never suggesting she might have doubts about my lagging recovery.

Waking each morning as the second week drew to a close, I no longer wondered when I would get out of the hospital. I had lost track of time in the fog of morphine, realizing only that I was here in a small ICU cubicle for an unknown amount of time.

GBS had its hold on me and no one was seeing any progress, not medical personnel nor my family. There was no point of reference to guide our expectations. No way to know when I might begin to move again. It was a game of wait-and-see with no end in sight.

Chapter Five

Learning to Cope

Remembering that first day in the emergency department, when doctors explained the course GBS was likely to take, I now had to admit it was clear I had fulfilled the whispered fears of worst case scenario that came only four days later. I realized I would have to set aside my hopeful thoughts of a quick recovery and begin learning to cope.

There was nothing left of the animated Carole who loved to walk the dogs or jog through the neighborhood. There was nothing left of the person who had walked briskly to work through bustling downtown crowds or played racket ball with her boss at lunch time. There was no one left to take active vacations with Stu or visit our children as they worked their separate pathways into adult life.

I was smothered in a blanket of fear. Why were we not seeing signs of the healing process that was supposed to start on its own? I kept forcing thoughts of permanent paralysis out of my mind because the neurologist assured us the process of GBS would reverse and I lay waiting. However, as night shadows gathered in the room and everyone else had gone home, the thought that this might never reverse itself came sneaking back.

A cheerful nurse swept into the room with a happy greeting. Her soft-soled shoes squeaked slightly as she approached the right side of the bed. She wound the blood pressure cuff around my upper arm and put a thermometer in my mouth. While she waited for results to register, she exchanged the empty plastic food bag that always dangled on the metal pole beside the bed.

I often pondered what it would be like to die in the midst of knowledgeable medical staff who were never aware I had needed their help. My heart raced unexpectedly at times. Gunk in my throat triggered fears of suffocating. The ventilator hose protruded from my neck and scrolled across the bedclothes to the machine at the side of the bed, a constant whirr helping me breathe. But what if someone dislodged the tube or accidently turned the ventilator off?

I wondered what Stu thought every time he walked into the room and saw me immobile, no progress to report. While he was always upbeat and hopeful, nothing seemed to change. Day after day I lay there, only my eyes blinking now and then to let him know I was still alive.

I have known Carole since we were both in eighth grade. We dated in high school, fell in love during our days in college, and truly appreciated our good fortune after we married and started our lives together.

Our relationship turned more serious in our senior year of high school as we planned for our future careers. My instinctive love for animals developed into thoughts of becoming a veterinarian. Carole's interests centered on political science and, although she never said so, the possibility of a career in law or politics. Carole wanted to get involved and make a difference.

We both chose Allegheny College, a small liberal arts school north of Pittsburgh, with an excellent pre-med program and a strong political science department.

As the school year began, Carole informed me our college years were a perfect time to date other people. It was a bruising revelation coupled with the college-wide announcement that she was the only freshman to make the cheerleading squad. This added to my dilemma of trying to keep Carole's interest as she was on display while I was banished to the role of a freshman nobody. Being a member of the football team helped a bit except for hearing the comments about how cute the new cheerleader was.

One day when no one else was around, kindly Dr. S arrived to exchange the Shiley in my trach. Shiley is the brand name of a device inserted into a tracheostomy to connect the patient's throat to a ventilator. He said he was here to replace my # 4 with a # 6.

The doctor's silver-grey hair and wire-rimmed glasses gave him a grandfatherly appearance as he prepared a tray of instruments and the device he would install in my neck. He worked efficiently and before I knew it, he held up the old Shiley and said the job was done.

As he looked down at me, a few tears fell from his eyes, rolled down his cheek and dropped silently onto my bed covers. I couldn't imagine why this simple procedure would make a doctor cry. Guessing I might wonder at this display of emotion over a simple Shiley replacement, he explained, "The last GBS patient I treated was during the Viet Nam War."

He went on to tell me, as a Navy physician, he had accompanied a stricken soldier out of the jungle in a medivac flight to Tokyo on Christmas Day. Guillain-Barré Syndrome had struck the soldier in the midst of war, reducing him to total paralysis. It must have been a moving experience for the young doctor, one he had carried with him to my bedside. Stu had served at the Naval Hospital at Quantico, Virginia during the Viet Nam war, causing me to consider whether our paths might have crossed with this doctor during those years. As I thought about the connection between the two of us, Dr. S turned quietly and walked out of my room.

One of the most frightening aspects of my time in the ICU was the possibility of contracting pneumonia. I heard conversations among physicians and nurses about GBS patients dying from lung infections before they could recover from GBS. "Oh, so that's what happens to some of the 20 percent who do not make a full recovery," I thought, hoping the respiratory therapists would be diligent in clearing my trach tube of secretions. Even with their careful attention, signs of infection appeared several times, prompting antibiotics and increased monitoring. I wondered if recurring infection was a bad sign.

If you've never been on a ventilator,* it's impossible to imagine how dependent you are on the respiratory therapists who cycle in and out of your life on the hospital's round-the-clock schedule. Some are sympathetic, carefully inserting the suction instrument into the trach tube that, of course, is attached to your throat. I worried about a careless slip puncturing my windpipe. These thoughtful therapists talk cheerfully and are efficient and purposeful in their treatment.

Others are rude, brusque, and careless. They rarely talk and if they do, it's to complain. Since suctioning occurs regularly throughout the day and night, it's impossible to avoid the bad ones or extend the service of the good ones. I only hoped to survive both.

Another necessary torture was the every-two-hour rollover to prevent bedsores. Nurses, accustomed to this procedure, quickly roll patients from back to side propping the new position with pillows, an easy maneuver for most patients to handle. But the extreme pain of GBS made those twelve "flips" a day pure agony for me. Like razorblades dragged over my skin, the nurses' hands prodded me to a new position. I endured these rollovers every time, praying for them to finish so my nerves could calm down to their regular pain level.

---

* Medical Appendix. Ventilators and Respirators.

A complication to this rolling procedure was the cumbersome boots wrapped around my feet to prevent foot drop, the debilitating collapse of muscles and tendons at the ankles. If not addressed early in a long hospitalization, a patient may be unable to walk even after extensive rehabilitation.

Fastened from heels to knees with Velcro, these boots with rigid bottoms held my feet perpendicular to my leg bones. They were clunky and if not positioned carefully, twisted my legs awkwardly at the hip joints. Few nurses ever seemed to think about my legs and feet when they rolled me. Perhaps some of them didn't know I was wearing the boots.

Once the roll was over and the pillows in place, they glided out of the room to the next patient not realizing my legs lay in a contorted jumble under the covers. I couldn't ask for help but only wait two hours for the next rollover when my legs might be straightened out.

Our compulsory separation lasted through first quarter, until Thanksgiving break when we returned home for a long weekend. To my amazement and pleasure, Carole agreed to go out with me while we were back on my home court.

The only details I remember about those dates were the great arguments about the whys and wherefores of dating in college – and an even greater reconciliation before we returned to campus fully committed to each other.

Every time I walked into her hospital room, in the unmoving husk on the bed I saw that effervescent college freshman wanting to come back to life.

While Dr. M devotedly tested for reflexes using the little rubber hammer, there were no reflexes for weeks; not one. Testing for strength, he slipped his fingers under each of my hands and said, "Squeeze my fingers, Carole."

I stared back with frustration and no voice and lay there inert, unable to comply. So, each morning I was reminded that my hands and arms were lifeless. This constant request to demonstrate strength was exceedingly frustrating although I realized it was important because, someday, there might be a small response showing that healing had begun. But, as each grindingly boring day went by, I questioned whether it would ever happen.

Paralysis of my eye muscles affected my sight. Hoping to help expand my world through reading, videos, and television Stu brought in a pair of glasses from home. Sadly, they could not compensate for the weakened eye muscles. I couldn't see well enough to read, but it wouldn't have mattered anyway because I couldn't turn the pages of a book. Watching videos or the television suspended above my bed would have been a marginally acceptable substitute, but to me the screen was a blurry smudge. I was devastated at this failed attempt to enlarge my world. What was I to do with these endless hours?

I knew while her body and its paralysis were the focus of everyone's attention, it was her mind and spirit that were under the greatest stress. To understand the woman who was now trapped within her own body only able to blink out brief messages, you have to understand the girl, the young lady, the mother, the publisher, the executive, the companion and wife.

I knew the soul of the person lying in that hospital bed staring at the ceiling. I knew her mind was full of questions. This was not an idle mind drifting from one aimless thought to another. This mind would be working overtime and would want to interact with those of us on the outside looking in.

Losing the ability to read was emotionally staggering. I shrank back into myself, music my only consolation and entertainment. Otherwise I had to rely on Stu, Eric, and Bonnie to bring me information, interpret medical jargon, and provide humor and stories to lift me out of myself. But there were so many hours in the day when none of them could be with me. If music wasn't playing, there was nothing but my small room, buzzing and clicking machines, and an occasional nurse or aide on a medical errand.

During the early weeks when Eric read the daily newspaper, I could focus on the topic, but as days went by and I slipped deeper into my own misery, my mind wandered as soon as he started to read. I found myself wanting the drone of his voice to stop. The pain in my bones tore my mind from the article and demanded that I think only of it. Mentally I felt like I was still deteriorating.

Stu stayed in touch with family members and friends, first letting them know about my condition, then providing periodic updates. But as days turned into weeks, he was overwhelmed by phone calls, emails, and written inquiries. Finally, in self-defense, Stu wrote the first of five *Carole's Chronicles*, a newsletter synopsis of my changing condition. A long-time friend set up a database of names and addresses from Stu's scribbled notes, then using Stu's draft, Linda printed Chronicle #1 and put it in the mail. None of us knew how many Chronicles would be necessary, but Linda was always available to send another as weeks of hospitalization stretched into months.

Day to day the routine was predictable. I awoke alone staring up at the grey vastness above me. I could see out to the bright light at the nurses' station and lay waiting for the parade of doctors and nurses, phlebotomists and respiratory therapists, aides and housekeepers to come to my room throughout the morning.

Stu stopped in for breakfast on his way to work, followed by Eric who put a CD in the player. As the room filled with music, I could close my eyes and relax, waiting for Eric to read the newspaper. The medical team came and went. When Eric left, Bonnie arrived. I listened to her stories of work, our sister, and mom. Then exhausted from doing nothing, I fell asleep, covered with the same light-weight white blanket as yesterday.

Small changes in this routine were welcome and stimulating. I always listened to new CDs brought by friends, hoping for something different to change my day. But invariably they all jolted my nerves and exhausted my patience. It seemed I could only tolerate classical music and Gregorian chants. Not knowing much about music theory or composition, I wondered what it was about those two styles of music that soothed me when no others did. I could listen to them for hours when a three-minute country music tune grated on my nerves.

Stu tried to keep most visitors away, but some people were undeterred. Dr. T, a long-time friend and compassionate doctor, seemed to know a brief visit could soothe and inspire. One day I awoke in mid-afternoon and looked up to see his head suspended just above my face with one hand on each side of my pillow. "Hi, Carole. It's Manny. I just came in to say hello and to tell you everything will get better." That was it: an unexpected change in a deadly boring routine that brightened the rest of the day.

Even more important were visits from family. While our children and Bonnie continued to visit regularly, my youngest sister Barbara and my mother were three hours away in Pittsburgh. It wasn't easy for them to make the trip and Stu undoubtedly told them I wouldn't be able to communicate. But now that several weeks had passed, they needed the reality of seeing me, in whatever condition, to help them understand what this disease is and how I was coping.

I will never forget them standing by the bed trying to take in all they were seeing. With my limited eyesight, they looked to me like two white discs with black eyes and red mouths floating in space next to the blinking heart monitor, the swaying bottle of IVIg fluid, and the beeping blood pressure monitor.

Even though Bonnie had explained my condition, it must have been devastating for them to see me as I was. I worried this would be too overwhelming for my mother, but she was tough. As Barbara talked quietly about their long drive to the hospital, Mom came close and gazed steadily into my eyes. I could almost hear her willing me to make the turn that would carry me to wellness while I was trying to share my thoughts about a brighter future with her.

While I wanted to sit up and hug her, we both knew that couldn't happen. We prolonged our mutual stare while Barbara and Stu conversed softly about what might happen next in my treatment. After a brief twenty-minute visit, Barbara moved to direct my mother out of the room. Mom deftly side-stepped the effort and bent over my bed, kissing me gently on the forehead. Then together they walked slowly out of the room.

I knew Carole's mind was not just lying idle. It couldn't be. It was thinking and struggling and absorbing every bit of stimulus it could get hold of. It was going to help Carole escape fully intact. God, I hoped so!

As I thought about Carole's personality and character during these difficult early days of her hospitalization, I considered what forces had made her the strong woman now totally immobile and silent in an ICU bed. Carole's father had been an Alcoa executive who traveled a great deal. His intellectual and inquisitive mind seemed to have been passed on to Carole.

After graduation from Allegheny, Carole achieved an MA in Education from the University of Michigan, eventually turning her education into a challenging job at the Columbus Area Chamber of Commerce as Vice President of Small Business and Government Affairs and a career as publisher and president of the city's business newspaper, Business First. *I hoped enough of that drive to succeed was still with her and she would use it now to fight her way back to the world she had left on Valentine's Day.*

Special interludes came rarely, so the day Stu announced it was time to make my college basketball March Madness picks, I was joyful. In years past, we had clipped the brackets from the daily paper and filled them in. This year Stu reproduced them on large sheets of paper and taped them to a blank wall in my ICU room, the huge black box letters visible even to me in bed just a few feet away.

With odds on each game in hand, Stu guided me through the match-ups, recording my picks alongside his. As the tournament proceeded, Stu noted the results of each game and posted them on his giant bracket sheet every evening. Word spread fast and soon interns and residents were popping in to check out the latest results. I loved listening to the wrangling about which teams were best and who would be the ultimate winner. Maybe my attention to this kind of detail was a sign of improvement?

The earliest glimmer of progress arrived in the form of a curly, dark-haired speech therapist who walked into my room one morning. Diana talked about what could be done to rejuvenate my speech and swallowing. I liked that she was positive, friendly, and upbeat. But what I liked best was that she talked directly to me rather than talking about me to others in the room as though I wasn't there.

Diana talked as though I was on the road to recovery and she was going to help me on that journey. But my mind reeled from the disconnect between her expectations for speech and eating when I was on a ventilator, couldn't talk, and hadn't eaten sold food for almost three weeks. Unable to hear my silent doubts, she continued with confidence, explaining how we would start by practicing moving my lips so later I'd be able to talk.

Hmmm? Practicing sounds without actually making them? It seemed a tricky proposition, but my dark-haired therapist just shook her curls, gave me a big smile and encouraged my cooperation. So, I thought, my lips must be moving enough for this exercise.

Every weekday Diana bounced into my room for a half-hour session, practicing lip formations. She also tested my swallowing reflexes and found them almost non-existent. But this told me, although she never said so, that some slight recovery was underway and we were preparing for what was to come. Even though small, this was the first bit of hope emerging from all these days of medical monitoring and edged me upward out of my pit of grinding despair.

But things still seemed dismal to me even if I could mouth an "O" or a "D". That seemed far from normal life and none of the rest of my body could move. I looked at my hands and willed just one finger to lift itself off the bed. Nothing. I tried to move my pelvis thinking that early signs of recovery might come from the core. Nothing there either. So, I tried to take speech therapy as a small first step toward further recovery.

My ability to breathe on my own was tested frequently, and by Day 25 the pulmonologist thought I was to the point where I might begin breathing on my own. He ordered the first trials off the ventilator. By placing me on oxygen through a mask rather than through the trach, they could begin conditioning my lungs for eventual return to breathing on my own.

This was a frightening prospect. I had grown dependent on the ventilator to breathe for me. Although I knew eventually I would work away from this dependence, I worried that my diaphragm wasn't strong enough. I wondered, if I couldn't get enough oxygen, would someone be there to reattach the ventilator to my trach? This fear was unwarranted. Over the next eight days, I increased my time off the ventilator from one to twelve hours, a monumental step. It meant there was improvement. The tide of Guillain-Barré Syndrome had reversed.

Chapter Six

The Asylum

One day without warning, my routine was scrambled immeasurably. After three weeks in the ICU, I was told I would be moving to a different hospital because OSU did not have a transitional unit to get me off the ventilator in preparation for aggressive therapy.

The head nurse explained that at the transitional hospital I would learn to sit up in a chair for two hours and be weaned from the ventilator before returning to OSU's Dodd Hall, home to its renowned physical therapy program. The impossibility of sitting up for two hours bounced around in my head, running into the facts of my current condition. My head moved only slightly. I couldn't talk. Or even sit up in bed yet. I wondered how long it would take to move from now to where they wanted me to be.

Then I was told I would travel this next phase of treatment without any of the doctors who had overseen my care at OSU's main medical campus. I tried to push back the fear of losing their oversight by assuring myself I must be making progress. Obviously, I no longer needed to be in the Intensive Care Unit. So, they were gently pushing me toward the next phase of treatment. "Progress," I told myself, but then whispered to myself, "But not much."

The ambulance was on standby as the nurses packed up my few personal possessions, my discharge papers, and me. While four nurses slid me from bed to a waiting gurney, Eric yanked the Western landscape from the ceiling. Stu rolled up the March Madness brackets, and the little white rag doll angel tagged along on my stomach as the staff gathered outside my room to say goodbye and good luck while the attendant released the brakes and pushed me toward the elevator.

As the EMT firmly slammed the ambulance doors shut behind us, I looked from side to side for a ventilator. I didn't see one and the EMT was fastening the gurney to the ambulance base, but not looking to connect me to a ventilator.

Fear grabbed me as I searched for rationality. "You know you can breathe on your own. You've done it for hours in the hospital." I closed my eyes and told myself to relax on the fifteen-minute ride to American Transitional Hospital (ATH), breathing slowly in and out, trying to keep a slow rhythm.

I thought about how I'd grown accustomed to the ICU routine. I recognized each nurse and therapist. I knew when my blood would be drawn, what time the speech therapist would show up, when the IVIg bottle would be hung. Now, I was headed to a different hospital with its own regimen and a new cast of characters. Would these people be as competent as those at the OSU main campus? Would they care as much about me? Would they know what to do to spur my recovery?

The wind was blowing hard when the ambulance pulled up to the emergency entrance of an incongruously round building. Quickly, as the gurney touched the ground, the EMTs, one on each side, rolled me toward the building. A corner of the blanket wrapped carefully around my head for protection against the wind whipped away and I savored the feeling of cold air on my face. After three weeks in the hospital, it was almost as good as a walk in the woods.

The automatic door sighed open and closed as we rolled into the hospital and glided toward a bank of elevators. The same kind of ceiling tiles that looked down at me in my room at OSU hung over me here: rows and rows of little black dots. Just as I focused in on them, bump, the gurney jostled over the elevator threshold and crashed into the left side rail.

No one spoke as the dull grey box of an elevator rose to the eighth floor where room 806 was ready for me. Two nurses and an aide slipped me off the gurney into a fresh bed. They attached the trach in my neck to a waiting ventilator and my anxiety subsided just a little bit.

Whoever thought of building a round hospital neglected to consider how difficult it would be to arrange furniture and equipment in a pie-shaped room. A large window was centered on the exterior wall allowing natural light to flood into the room: a nice upgrade from the windowless ICU. The facing wall is about twice as wide as the extra-large door opening into the hallway, leaving the remaining two oblique walls to anchor medical equipment, a small table, and a chair or two.

While I cased out the room and mentally chastised the architect who came up with such an unlikely configuration, a team of nurses and aides prepared me to morph from an ICU patient to a transitional one. Ruthann, the head nurse, took my vital signs, jotting them down on the raft of paper she carried on a brown clipboard. I guessed her to be about 5' 4" tall, in excellent physical condition and with a take-charge demeanor softened by her quiet voice, attention to detail, and willingness to take time for brief side comments that put me at ease.

Ruthann flipped up the top page to check the notes that had come with me from OSU and proposed changing the feeding tube running through my left nostril into my stomach. It had been placed almost three weeks prior and should have been exchanged by now for a Percutaneous Endoscopic Gastronomy (PEG).*

The notes told the nurse the first time a physician at OSU had attempted to place a PEG, it was discovered I had hemorrhagic gastritis as well as pancreatitis so they aborted the effort. Here at ATH they checked the condition of my stomach and found I still had gastritis. The doctor was consulted and determined to leave the nose tube while monitoring the condition of my stomach and, perhaps, placing the PEG later.

Following doctor's orders, Ruthann deftly pulled the old tube up and out of my nose, wrapped it in a paper towel and dropped it lightly on the elevated tray positioned to the right of the bed. As she prepared to insert the new one, I glanced at what had to go back through my nose and into my stomach. The clear, flexible tube looked incredibly large. I closed my eyes and elevated my chin as Ruthann proved her expertise with a quick insertion. I had confidence in her already.

After taping the protruding end of the tube to the side of my face, Ruthann hung a bag of liquid nourishment just out of view to the right rear of the bed. She then swiftly attached heart monitors, inserted a catheter, and placed an IV in my right arm. I was amazed how efficiently she accomplished these tasks all the while talking quietly to me about how they would take good care of me here.

I had been free of wires and tubes for about an hour, but now things looked pretty much as they had at OSU. The atmosphere, though, was not as somber as in the ICU and my spirit lightened a little as I anticipated making progress in this new environment.

* * *

---

* Medical Appendix. Percutaneous Endoscopic Gastronomy (PEG)

As time went on I learned the personalities and quirks of all the nurses who would attend me for what turned out to be a two-month stay. The two most regular nurses, Ruthann on days and Jayme on the evening shift, were so reassuring that I was always glad when they were on duty. The night shift nurses and those who filled in on weekends seemed remote and less caring. I found it difficult to establish rapport with them because they always seemed to be hurrying somewhere else.

Just like the rough respiratory therapists and night nurses I feared at OSU, there were people at ATH who should not be working there. Shortly after my arrival, a nurse walked briskly into the room. I heard her enter, but she was out of my sight until she suddenly leaned over the bed, a hand on each side of my pillow, her face about two inches above mine and hissed a warning. "I don't want any trouble out of you or I can make things very rough." Totally shocked, I wondered what kind of asylum I'd entered.

Perhaps because of my medications, how close she was to me when she delivered her message, or my utter surprise, I was never able to conjure an image of her face. As soon as she finished warning me, she turned abruptly and hurried out of the room. I noticed she had medium brown hair pulled back in a long ponytail, but I never could identify her during my long stay at ATH.

Years later I read a doctor's note in my medical record. It said I "was quite demanding on the staff although very good care was rendered." No one ever spoke to Stu about this. Nor did I get the impression from other nurses or aides that I was particularly demanding. It made me wonder if that threatening nurse had the doctor's ear.

The only episode I remember that may have labelled me as a troublesome patient was when friends Larry and Kay unexpectedly walked into my room my first full day at ATH. It was a quiet time when no one else was around. They lived not too far from the hospital, had heard I was being transferred, and decided to stop by to say hello.

Thin and fit, Larry bounded through the door first. His khaki pants and blue Oxford shirt made him look like a graduate student although he was a senior partner at one of the city's preeminent architectural firms. Kay was as enthusiastic as Larry, her honey colored curls swinging with her bouncy walk. They both acted like I was sitting up waiting for a chat even though no words were coming out of my mouth, my hair had been unwashed for three weeks, I had a plastic bag of ice on my head, and a gastric tube taped to my face. Yet, Larry and Kay tuned in right away to reading my lips. Larry asked if there was anything I needed.

It was March, still cold in Central Ohio. The temperature in the hospital was set at an appropriate level, but GBS had affected my autonomic nervous system* in a way that caused me to feel excessively warm. That morning, I was burning up even with the ice bag on my forehead. I suggested that a fan might help cool me off.

Larry and Kay headed home, returning with a fan which they attached to the foot of the bed directing the breeze toward my face. Even though it was small, the fan created a gentle breeze. The ruffle of air felt wonderful – but only for a brief time. A nurse soon entered and told us this type of fan was not permitted. This was not the efficient, caring Ruthann, but rather a large drill sergeant in white nurse's uniform. "This fan doesn't have the correct URL rating," she insisted.

After determining what kind of fan would be acceptable, Kay and Larry left in search of a better fan. Returning with a larger model, the proper URL label attached, Larry beamed, "Let's see how this one works." It, too, was firmly rejected.

Abandoning the fan idea, the three of us chatted amiably until the drill sergeant-nurse showed up accompanied by a technician carrying a very large, standing fan. It was about five feet tall and quite heavy. In my small room there was little space for such a monstrous fan but, with Larry's help, the technician found a space.

When the nurse flipped the switch, a gale force wind blew as the blades rattled in their metal casement. She dialed back the speed to a comfortable setting, but the whole effort was way out of proportion to my needs. The fan stayed in my room, unused until a week later when someone finally removed it.

* * *

The medical staff was an invisible factor in my care at ATH. The day I arrived, I never saw a physician. Nor on any of the following sixty days. The nurses would say, "I'll check that with the doctor." Or, "Dr. R will have to consider what to do about that." Yet, Dr. R never once appeared at my bedside.

The repercussions of this lack of oversight were devastating. No doctor came to check my reflexes as Dr. M had done at OSU. While that routine was frustrating when I couldn't move at all, now it would have informed the doctor

---

* Medical Appendix. Autonomic and Somatic Nervous Systems

of the first glimmer of movement in my fingers. It also would have given him a baseline to measure my progress, and given me the comforting anticipation of recovery.

The second example of lack of attention or misunderstanding of continuity of care wasn't obvious until I returned to OSU two months later. The two courses of IVIg administered in the ICU seemed to instigate some small gains: return of facial tone, slight movement of my head; a weak smile and the ability to move my lips. But there were no IVIg treatments administered to me at ATH. So, for two months I did not receive therapy that could have accelerated my recovery. The physician in charge mentions these treatments in his admission notes, but never prescribed any more while I was under his care. Forever I will wonder why not.

In his admission notes Dr. R wrote that the "ultimate goal" is to prepare me for rehabilitation at OSU. He mentions the trach collar trials as a positive, notes previous infections which are no longer evident, yet never mentions pain at all. This was the third and most devastating example of this physician's ignorance of my symptoms and his treatment of Guillain-Barré Syndrome. The doctors at OSU understood that pain can be a significant factor for GBS patients and treated my pain aggressively. An understanding of my intense pain was devastatingly missing at ATH. But it shouldn't have been. This brief extract from a nursing textbook explains the pain issue clearly:

> "About 25% of patients will experience pain. Pain is underrated in terms of *frequency and intensity.* (Emphasis mine.) The pain may begin as cramping and progress to frank (meaning clinically evident) pain in the arms, legs, back, or buttock. Pain is often worse at night and often interferes with sleep. Analgesics are often necessary to keep the patient comfortable. The pain may be so severe that a morphine drip is necessary." (Degenerative Diseases of the Nervous System, p. 653) Further, this text notes, *"The quality and quantity of the pain and fear associated with the acute phase of GBS are unique to this illness.* (Emphasis mine.)

Dr. R also reflected in my medical record his concern about my high level of anxiety. On the day I was transferred from OSU he noted, "Mrs. Williams did well after arrival to ATH, although her mental status remained one of her major problems."

Almost a month later when I was being propped in a chair for long periods of time, Dr. R acknowledged that "Pain control became an issue as she began to eventually develop recovery of her neurological deficits." This is completely incorrect. I had excruciating pain from the outset of this disease. It did not just come on as I started to recover. He never believed what he heard from Stu or from the nurses about the pain I was experiencing and wrote in the medical record that he refused to increase the amount of anxiety medication I was receiving and "she will just have to learn to deal with it."

By the first week in April, Dr. R's views had not changed. He had not made the connection between extreme pain and high anxiety. He wrote, "...she is doing relatively well with her mental status being a continuing major factor inhibiting her recovery. She remained extremely anxious." *

While recovery from GBS is primarily a physical process, a patient's mental condition has to be entered into the equation. Constant, unrelenting pain does cause anxiety. It interferes with concentration during therapy. It nags during morning rounds and in the quiet afternoons. It throbs when the night nurses come to roll you over, take your temperature, or adjust your monitors.

There is never a moment without pain, just more or less of it. It would have helped my "mental status" to have the proper type and level of medication to reduce the pain and, thus, lower my anxiety.

I see this as total medical ignorance and incompetence. It is questionable, in my mind, whether this doctor was well acquainted with Guillain-Barré Syndrome, its epidemiology, clinical presentation and recommended course of treatment. Given the cranky nurse, Dr. R, and others I was yet to meet, I sometimes wondered who was running this asylum.

---

* Medical Appendix. Pain and Anxiety

Chapter Seven

Range of Motion

A *s I stood at the foot of her bed, I realized there was no way the staff at ATH could begin to appreciate Carole's personality, warmth, and intelligence. Just as in the ICU, I wanted to help them understand her, so the next day, I hung my favorite picture of Carole at the head of the bed, her name written on a piece of white paper taped to the bottom of the frame.*

Some staff wondered aloud whose picture it was, but the majority got the message immediately without realizing there had been a problem. The picture quietly made the point that the GBS patient in room 806 was a human being with a smile and a personality. I believe it made a difference in how nurses, therapists, aides and, yes, even physicians related to her.

When Diana encouraged me in the odd exercise of making the shapes of sounds in the ICU, I hadn't realized she was an ATH speech therapist on loan to OSU. So, it was a happy surprise when she came into my room on Monday to continue our silent lip gymnastics. The twenty-minute daily routine still seemed somewhat absurd, making me wonder every day when I would actually be able to talk.

Although a tedious exercise, speech therapy was easy compared to the new routine of occupational and physical therapy. Three weeks of not moving was about to end for me and Phyllis, the best aide imaginable, explained the daily routine we were going to follow.

"Every weekday morning therapists will exercise your arms and legs. I'm going to get you ready by warming up your muscles with heating pads."

I dreaded the thought of people moving my arms and legs. Because even a light touch on my arm sent cascades of pain through my body, I couldn't imagine making regular, sustained movement of any kind. But I had to accept that this was the beginning of my rehabilitation and I had to prepare myself mentally for a long and difficult struggle.

They wasted no time. Monday through Friday, Ruthann gave extra pain medication first thing in the morning in anticipation of the coming workout. As the pain medication took effect, Phyllis, a large woman with a jovial demeanor interwoven with a professional attitude let me know, "You will work hard to help yourself recover and I'm going to make sure you do that," as she came into my room with a cart full of hot, muscle-relaxing pads.

With the tearing sound of Velcro, she gingerly removed my awkward knee-high boots and set them on the floor next to the wall. Then she gingerly placed the warm pads, wrapping them around my joints and over the long muscles of my legs and arms, chatting all the while. The heat penetrated the sheet and cotton blanket and worked its way into my arms, hands, and legs. The soothing warmth reminded me of those hot showers I took during the onset of GBS. Heat definitely helped ease the pain.

Phyllis flashed a cheerful smile and left me to warm up for a half hour. As she walked out the door, she always left me with a message, "See you later." Or, "Try to relax. They'll be here in a little while." I closed my eyes and enjoyed the brief respite before what I knew would be a grueling, painful workout.

The physical therapist arrived first. A brief smile flitted across her Asian features as Yero greeted me and prepared to work. Her long black hair sparkled from the overhead fluorescents and swung from side to side as she removed the heating pads from one leg to begin stretching it with a bend at each joint. First the hip. She raised my left leg as far as she could push it toward my head, applying pressure to stretch the taut muscles.

Despite the additional medication, the pain was excruciating. I couldn't scream. I couldn't retract my leg. My muscles and physical reflexes had failed me, leaving me alone with the pain. I squeezed my eyes shut, trying to envision the hamstring muscle stretching. Yero held my leg in place while, teeth gritted, I stood the pain through her long count...18...19...20. Release. I mentally sank back into my pillow, gathering myself for the next stretch.

Yero's objective was to give me as much range of motion* as possible. The term "range of motion" was one I was to hear every day. I learned that every part of my body needed to be stretched beyond what I ever thought possible –

---

* Medical Appendix. Range of Motion

first to maintain what range of motion I had and then gradually to increase that range – always working toward what I used to have before I was felled by GBS.

When she finished with both hips, Yero moved to the knees. The procedure was similar: a stretch to my current range of motion, hold for a count of twenty, then repeat. The tendons around my knees were so tight, they seemed to be frozen straight out with no bend at all. Yero fought the constrictions in those tendons trying to get a little more flexibility each day.

Next, she tackled the ankles. While the monster boots held my feet perpendicular to my shins when I was resting in bed, Yero now worked those ankles in every direction trying to recreate flexibility that was almost totally gone.

Yero moved quickly from one exercise to the next, trying to get to all the joints in her allotted time. This stretching didn't require any participation on my part, letting me focus on the good feeling of heat in my arms and hands to minimize the bad feeling of pain in my legs.

When she was done with the second leg, Yero strapped the boots back on, waved "Goodbye" and hurried on to her next patient.

As soon as the physical therapist finished, two occupational therapists came into the room. One worked on my arms while the other focused solely on my hands. While work on the legs was extremely painful, what needed to be done on my hands caused so much pain, I have no words to describe it.

Years after the experience I have no recollection of the woman who worked on my arms and shoulders, but the hand specialist's face is locked in my permanent memory. A young woman of average height, Gina pulled back an abundance of long, curly, strawberry blond hair with a clip on the top of her head. She smiled and chatted and shared her knowledge of hand rehabilitation as she worked diligently on me.

The first day she explained,

> "Let's look at your hands and think about the number of joints we have to work on. Three joints in each finger and other joints in the hand itself. We're going to work every joint every day to be sure you have use of your hands when you are finally well."

True to her word, every day Gina manipulated each joint in each hand. Knowing how much pain I was in, she always talked about the importance of getting full function back in my hands and that it was necessary to endure the pain to succeed. I knew she was right but I still cried my way through every session. And because we had no sessions on weekends, Gina showed Stu and

Eric the procedures and told them how important it was to continue these exercises on Saturdays and Sundays.

Gina was the second person who encouraged me to think of the day when I would be totally back to normal. Like Diana, every time I saw her, she renewed my hope of getting well and she made me see the importance of working through the pain to that end.

Compared to the hand therapy, work on my arms seemed easy and much less painful. While Gina worked on the left hand, the other therapist worked on the right arm. Then they changed places and went through the same routine again. I concentrated on the hand therapy, looking at the strawberry blond curls and willing myself to remember we were both working toward my future.

At the end of the first week in April, Dr. R noted in my chart that he was going to increase my pain medication because at this stage of my recovery I was "beginning to experience more pain." From inside the body that had borne this pain for five weeks, I could have told him that, indeed, I was experiencing more pain because of the therapy. But I also could have told him the pain of Guillain-Barré Syndrome is excruciating and never ending. It started four days before I was diagnosed and had never let up, no matter what he thought.

While I was relieved when therapy ended, the rest of the boring day loomed ahead of me. Now that I was in less danger than I was in the ICU, Stu, Eric, and Bonnie spent a little less time with me. Because I still couldn't read or watch television, I closed my eyes and thought of my future and what I had to do to get there before falling asleep, exhausted.

In the late afternoon, I listened to the sounds of hospital bustle flowing in my door from the eighth-floor corridor. The gentleman next door was definitely unhappy and was very vocal about his distress. I could hear him yelling to the nurses,

"Come and get me out of this bed. I'm going to pull out my IVs if you don't come now."

Soon a nurse's voice called back to him from a distance,

"You can't get out of bed, John, you have a catheter in." As soon as the nurse stopped talking, he called out again that he wanted to get out of bed.

This went on for hours every afternoon and early evening. Finally, he would quiet down and go to sleep only to start up again the next day with the same plaintive calls.

I thought a lot about another patient who was admitted a week or so after I was. This young woman had had a brain hemorrhage during a normal delivery following a normal pregnancy. Irreversible damage had been done and she was at ATH while her family decided their best course of action. Although I never saw her or members of her family, Stu filled me in on the sad details of this tragedy, and I often lay in bed thinking of her and the devastation that came to this young family out of nowhere.

There was a brand new, healthy baby; a young sibling; a grief-stricken husband, and her devastated parents. This woman would never get off the ventilator, never walk out of this hospital, never hold her new baby or live life again. It made me grateful that although I was still mostly paralyzed, I might be able to work my way back to health and return to my former life.

The lady in the room to the left of mine had had a stroke. She would have to endure physical therapy and the process of getting off the ventilator just as I would. We had that in common and something else that developed over time – the interest and support of her son.

One day he stuck his head in my door and asked if he could come in. With a nod, I agreed. I don't know how he came to know my story, but he was just like Kay and Larry in his ability to understand the formation of my words rather than having to hear them.

When I saw that round, smiling face topped with a bright-colored cap, peek around the door frame, I was happy to see him. He started each visit with something cheerful then gave me an update on his mother's progress and asked about mine. It felt like we were having a conversation even though it was one-sided.

One day he approached the bed and asked if he could pin a small square of red and yellow cloth on my hospital gown. I nodded and with a standard safety pin he affixed the prayer cloth telling me all the people in his church were praying for me. This touched me deeply and remains a symbol in my memory of all the hundreds of people who did so much to support me spiritually and emotionally for more than a year through all my trials.

A nurse from the fifth floor had heard there was a Guillain-Barré patient on the eighth floor and came by to share her experience with me. She came into the room quietly and stood watching me. She was a large woman, tall and broad with a kindly face and sad looking eyes. Long black hair hung to her shoulders. I thought how capable she looked and imagined that she would be a comforting and very able nurse.

She explained that she had been fighting her own battle with GBS for about a year and had recently returned to work. This gave me confidence that I, too, might be able to return to an active life. But a year of recuperation was way outside what I had been anticipating. My heart sank even further when she asked, "Do you mind if I sit down while we talk?" as she retrieved a wheelchair from out of my sight. "So," I thought, "after a yearlong struggle, she still needs a wheelchair." This was a stab of reality that after a very long battle against GBS the result might be something less than a full recovery.

She told me some stories about her own illness and recovery -- enough to be encouraging without revealing all the pain and hard work it was going to require to get me to where she was. She shared several ideas about how to cope in a fight against GBS. The best and most practical was to hang a large calendar on the wall where nurses and family members could make notes about my progress. She knew progress seems excruciatingly slow when it's happening but that each day brings new achievements. By detailing these little bits of progress, the path to larger achievements seems more obvious. I was enjoying the interaction so much that, at first, I didn't notice she was crying. When she was unable to control her tears any longer, she quickly spun the wheelchair in a tight circle, waved goodbye and rolled out of the room.

Nurses in the ICU had gradually begun the weaning process weeks ago by methodically reducing the pressure on the ventilator for short periods each day allowing Carole to breathe on her own. A little at a time, she gained back strength in her chest. Now it was time to push harder to break her dependence on the ventilator.

Barbara F, one of the most attentive respiratory therapists, wanting to prepare Carole for the final push to get off the ventilator, approached with a confident smile and said,

> *"Carole, this morning you're going to have your first trial totally off the ventilator."*

> *"You mean without the trach mask," I voiced Carole's obvious concern.*

> *"Yes, she's ready to do it. And I'll be right here."*

Carole took a last artificial breath as Barbara, switched the knob to "off." Carole's dark eyes blinked rapidly as she concentrated on every aspect of breathing. I could imagine her mind saying,

> *"In, out, in, out. Expand your chest. Concentrate. In, out."*

> *"Keep going. You're doing great," I said, holding back a flood of emotion.*

With determination in her eyes, Carole raised her left hand slightly off the bed, a gesture that a few weeks ago would have been impossible. Both the look in her eyes and her hand signal told Barbara we were going longer than two minutes.

"Okay, Carole," Barbara agreed. A moment later she said,

"That was a notch over three minutes. Nice work! I'm glad you pushed for the extra time. We'll do this several times a day from now on and you'll be off this machine before you know it."

As she settled back on a pile of pillows, a mixture of relief, satisfaction, triumph, and joy came over Carole's face. Her feelings surely reflected my own.

Stark memories flashed through my mind. The morning we awoke to her paralysis from the knees down. The day she was placed on the ventilator, cutting our communication to zero. The Saturday after her admission when the only movement and the only Carole I could see was the look in her eyes. The motionless days in the ICU. Today was significant. Carole was on her way back.

Chapter Eight

Friends and Enemies

I settled into the ATH routine during the work week as Stu, Eric, and Bonnie continued their faithful rotation. Glen visited when he could get away from work and Katie and Keith drove back from Allegheny almost every weekend.

Stu continued to limit my visitors, a very good idea, but people came nonetheless. My boss made regular visits, staying fifteen minutes each time, talking mostly about the health systems' merger and how much she wished I were there to help. Trying to glance sideways to engage in the conversation, I caught the image of Sandy, trim and fit, her straight, sandy brown hair cut at a medium length.

As she talked, I thought warmly of our work together and our contests on the racket ball court. I could read the pain she felt for me in her face and wished I could reassure her that I was making progress. My sympathy flowed back to her as I knew the huge project she was talking about could easily overwhelm our medium-sized firm. Yet, it looked like I wouldn't be out of the hospital any time soon to help.

One person who continued to show up regularly was our treasured friend, the OSU professor we had met years ago in Ann Arbor. He was in constant contact with Stu while I was in the ICU, making my cubicle a regular stopping off point during his days on campus.

Now that I was many miles from the university campus, Steve still stopped by several times a week. When that tan, craggy face topped with wavy silver hair popped into my room, I knew his ever-present smile and upbeat conversation would entertain and encourage me.

After talking with me for a while he would say goodbye, put an arm around Stu's shoulders and guide him out into the hallway. I hoped Steve was giving Stu even more support than he was giving me. I knew Stu was being dragged down by the lack of progress I was making. Surely the burden of paying for this care was also weighing on his mind. And I knew he must have doubts about whether I would ever recover at all. Maybe Steve's quiet compassion could help where I couldn't.

Parting with Carole every evening was tough. I would kiss her on the forehead and look into her eyes. I wasn't sure what I saw. Was it relaxation after a rough day of therapy? Or was it the anxiety of another long, lonesome night? I just couldn't tell. I longed for her to talk again. To move and sing and walk. But none of this was happening.

One evening, as I walked to my car, the raw emotions I had buried since Valentine's Day rushed to the surface. I could feel them slipping out right there as I crossed a small grassy area sprinkled with a light dusting of snow. Just as the first tear rolled down my cheek, I heard Steve L, call out,

"Stu, is that you? Wait up. How's Carole doing?"

I turned, and just as he reached me, a cascade of tears fell. I couldn't say a word. Steve grabbed me in a strong bear hug and just let me cry for a while.

When we did speak, I explained that while Carole was now at the transitional hospital, she was still 95 percent paralyzed and in considerable pain. No one could tell us if she could gain back everything she had lost. I admitted I was scared to death and was beginning to understand the saying, "fear of the unknown."

Steve spoke few words that evening, but did give me reassurance and comfort, as he would on many occasions in the next several months. I valued his compassion and quiet reassurance.

Other people stopped by when I was sleeping. Some left notes on the bedside table. Several mailed handwritten letters to the hospital where each one was read to me. Like so much else about recovering from GBS, the impact of all that goodwill was incremental and didn't hit me until years later when I sat down and read three grocery bags full of notes, letters, cards, and articles.

Each message helped lift my spirits, but just like a tiny bit of physical progress in my fight against GBS, it was hardly noticeable until I looked back over time and appreciated how each bit added up to an enormous amount of caring.

One visitor surprised Stu and me more than anyone else when he arrived around 5:30 one evening. Carrying a potted plant, the Ethiopian parking lot attendant walked quietly into my room. He extended the plant toward Stu and whispered a few words about hoping I would get well soon. Lying in bed, unmoving, I wondered how he had found out what had happened to me, how he knew which hospital I was in, and how he found his way here after work.

I knew only a little about him. He had come to the United States from Africa, hoping to build a better life for himself. He worked at the parking lot every day, hoping to save enough money so his family could join him. Such a lonely existence propelled solely with hope for the future. I didn't even know his full name.

In his quiet way, after a few minutes, he said, "Goodbye," and walked out of my room, leaving me to marvel at what caring was in his heart to make him take the time to find me and share his thoughts that day. Stu looked at me in wonder. Certainly, he had no idea who this person was and I couldn't explain.

Unexpected surprises were rare at ATH but when they did arrive, they added a sparkle of joy to an otherwise pretty boring routine. One afternoon several aides offered me an impromptu tour of the eighth floor. I nodded in joyful anticipation.

Trach mask in place, they disconnected me from the ventilator, then swung the bed toward the door. Down the hall we went. Finally, I could see all of the people I had been imagining in my mind.

I peeked in the room of the stroke patient next door. She was napping. The next two rooms were occupied with wide awake patients so we stopped for introductions and one-sided chats.

On around the circular hallway we rolled and as we came near my room, I got a look at the patient who yelled every afternoon for the nurse to take out his IV. His white wispy hair stuck out in all directions. The sheets were rumpled and his right leg dangled over the edge of the bed. The quick wave he gave when introduced, showed me his happy side. He wasn't an ogre, just a nice little old man who wanted to go home.

✳ ✳ ✳

Now that I was awake for longer periods of time, ventilator-assisted breathing seemed much more challenging. Often, I felt an overwhelming choking sensation as my throat clogged with mucous, the very reason respiratory therapists regularly suction ventilator patients. I felt like I was drowning.

Once my head was mobile, I was given a flat, circular call button that rested on my pillow. With a roll of my head, I could call a nurse if I needed assistance. Reassuring, unless no one responded.

Because response time varied widely, I always faced a thought-provoking choice. When I began to feel distress, I wondered whether I should wait for it to get worse so I wouldn't bother them or to call early to give the respiratory therapist time to reach me before I slipped into panic mode.

Usually I hit the right balance, but there was one episode that showed me nurses might not always pay attention to the monitors. One night I felt discomfort breathing and waited for some time to see if the problem would resolve itself. It didn't. Instead, it grew worse. And worse. I felt for the call button with my head. It was out of reach.

Panic enveloped me. The constriction in my throat was acute. I could take in very little air. My heart was beating much too fast. I could think of nothing but suffocating in this hospital bed with no one around to help. My heart beat faster and faster. I felt trills and irregular heartbeats. I forced myself to stay calm, but finally, I couldn't get any breath at all. No one came.

More excruciating minutes passed before an aide wandered in. I shook my head rapidly from side to side trying to signal a need for help. Seeing my distress, she called for a respiratory therapist and within minutes I had been suctioned and was beginning to calm down.* My racing heart retuned slowly to normal.

The messages I blinked out to Stu the next day give a stark picture of what I experienced.

"Last night was terrifying." Then,

"Missed suction. Didn't know what to do."

Stu asked, "Do you want to talk with the doctor so he can talk with the nurse and therapist?"

I replied, "I think she (the respiratory therapist) will take it out on me." Trying to be a comfort, Stu asked,

"Do you want me to stay tonight?"

While I wished someone could be with me all the time to protect me from actions I couldn't control, it was unreasonable to expect Stu to do that. I blinked out,

---

* Medical Appendix. Respiratory Therapists and the Suctioning Procedure

"Let's see how things go today."

And that's what we did. We let it go.

GBS is a terrifying experience. Many healthcare workers know little about it and seem to be making up their treatment ideas as they go along which gives little comfort to patients and their families who search wherever they can for information. Our friends and family searched the Internet and talked with as many people as possible to find out about this condition.

A nurse friend gave us an insight into her training on working with patients on ventilators. The clip she chose said:

> "Most (GBS) patients are very fearful, communicating the ultimate fear, a fear of dying....To be fully conscious and cognitively intact yet be on ventilatory support must be an overwhelmingly frightening experience. Some patients are maintained on a ventilator for a few months before weaning is completed and need much information and continued support throughout the long months of recovery."

At the time, I thought it was just my own experience with breathing difficulties that caused anxiety, a personal problem. But this is common in many GBS patients on a ventilator as this nursing textbook confirms: "Respiratory insufficiency can cause anxiety."

One thing Dr. R may have suggested to ameliorate my anxiety was religious consultation. I don't know if it was his idea, but in my medical record I found pastoral notes showing attempts to overcome my anxiety.

One disheveled gentleman arrived unannounced at my bedside late in the afternoon. After introducing himself, he straightened his suitcoat, walked to the side of my bed and took a seat then read a brief passage of scripture, rose from the chair and excused himself. After three similar visits, he never returned.

Then a female religious person showed up. She seemed ill at ease, staring over my head and never looking at me as she tried to talk consolation and uplift. Scripture and prayer were not in her repertoire and with no response from me, she may have been totally frustrated. She left quickly, never to return.

I would have welcomed help from either of these well-meaning people, but neither acknowledged knowing I was anxious. Instead, they simply left me wondering if anyone had explained to them what GBS is, how I was being treated, and the prognosis so they could talk optimistically with me.

The most helpful religious support was direct contact from people who had attended church with us in the past or people with deep religious conviction who wrote me supportive notes. Just thinking about people caring enough to find the right poem, article, or book to provide comfort was supportive beyond what they could imagine.

Another small surprise came when the nurses and therapists decided on a sunny March day to take me on a "walk" outside the hospital. I don't know who thought of it, but she knew more about lowering anxiety than the physician and the religious folks combined.

Yero, the physical therapist, brought three extra blankets and bundled me up from my ungainly boots to my chin like a giant winter coat without sleeves. Down we went in the elevator and out the door into a sunny, breezy spring day. Three people kept me company on a short stroll on the sidewalk until we reached a fountain in a small, landscaped garden.

American Transitional Hospital is in an urban area with very little outside space, but someone thought enough of staff, patients, and families to design a pleasing oasis amid concte and traffic. Water splashed down the core of the nine-foot fountain, burbling and gurgling while the sun peeped through stark grey tree branches warming my face as I stared up into the bluest of skies.

❊ ❊ ❊

Shortly after my arrival at ATH, E. coli was discovered in my sputum. Evidently, though I wasn't aware, the gunk suctioned from my throat was analyzed in the laboratory regularly. This infection interfered with attempts to begin weaning me off the ventilator and also made it more difficult for me to breathe. The infection was monitored with X-rays taken on the night shift.

Just like some nighttime respiratory therapists, some nighttime X-ray technicians can be brutal. The one I remember most vividly rattled into my room around 3:00 am with his equipment and X-ray plates jangling on a rolling cart. As he woke me from a sound sleep he announced, "Here to take an X-ray, " then grabbed my hospital gown with his huge fist, pulling me up and forward off the bed. After slapping a large X-ray film on the bed, he dropped me back onto the cold plate sending cascades of pain through my body.

It was a long fall from an upright sitting position down to the icy cold metal and glass plate. The edges were sharp and if he didn't drop me squarely in the right spot, a couple of ribs, my pelvis, or an elbow hit the edge of the plate. Another growl, another grab and hoist. Another drop onto the plate. Where do people like this come from?

✳ ✳ ✳

The primary goal of the ATH staff was to get me off the ventilator and breathing on my own. At the same time, through speech therapy, they were working to prepare me to speak again and educating me about what I needed to do to begin eating on my own. Along with aggressive therapy, the second goal was to change me from an unmoving, reclined patient to one who could sit up on her own.

Eighteen days after admission to ATH, Ruthann told me I was going to sit up for the first time in five weeks. As several therapists and aides looked on, she explained the process,

> "We're going to raise you to a sitting position, turn your body so your legs hang over the side of the bed and let you sit there for a minute or two."

"Don't worry," Diana offered, "We're all here to help."

It sounded so easy, but my mind was screaming the impossibility of it. I feared the hose connecting me to the ventilator would be dislodged. I knew I couldn't support myself and would be relying on other people to hold me stable on the edge of the bed. Visions of my body sliding off the bed and crashing to the floor filled my mind. And the pain of all that movement, I knew, would be unbearable.

Everyone was understanding, as if they could read my thoughts, but also gently forceful in letting me know today was the beginning of learning to sit up and we were going to proceed whether I thought I was ready or not.

Everyone took their places around the bed. With a touch of her foot, Ruthann set the bed whirring and clicking. The head of the automatic bed rose slowly toward perpendicular, causing panic to rise in my throat. I felt like I was going to topple forward folding over myself. But Diana supported me on my right side and Gina on my left. They chatted about what an important step this was for me and assured me they would not let me fall.

Yero and Phyllis, propped me up from behind, their hands on each shoulder. An aide straightened the ventilator hose as we made each move and held it out from my throat to keep it from kinking. Then Phyllis and Yero pulled my shoulders farther forward as Ruthann swung my legs off the bed, letting them drop over the side. Like a rag doll unable to control any of my own movements, I swayed from side to side. But steady hands held me.

I felt myself smiling inside although I couldn't show much feeling on the outside. I looked at my legs dangling toward the floor. Yep, I still had legs. I couldn't feel them, but everyone said I would be strong enough in a few months to start learning how to walk. It seemed impossible but this first time being upright gave me the hope that it was true.

I realized I was holding my head up by myself. I looked from side to side enjoying the happy expressions on everyone's faces. Dizzy and a bit disoriented, I was able to stand the strain for about two minutes when, as promised, they gently lowered me back into bed. I felt a flood of happiness wash over me. It was like running a 5K race even though it was only sitting up for two minutes. It felt amazing.

Chapter Nine

Returning Function

The boring therapy routine continued day after day with little variation. Each weekday morning Phyllis wrapped me in soothing hot packs and left me to toast until the therapists arrived. While I waited for Yero to take a more aggressive approach with my legs, I wondered why therapy on my feet wasn't as thorough as on my hands. Certainly, if I was to walk again, working the muscles and tendons in my feet was essential. By evening, when I had a chance to formulate a blinked message about this, I couldn't think how to explain my concerns in a brief way, so I never did. I just continued to wonder.

On the flip side, hand therapy was more aggressive every day. As the third week at ATH began, Gina gave me specially constructed gloves to wear after each day's grueling therapy. Made of tan mesh, the gloves had rubber bands attached to the tips of each finger and thumb. Gina maneuvered the gloves onto my hands, then stretched each rubber band tightly, attaching them to the wrist hook. The stretch ran over my wrists and across the top of my hands, a pull so strong it felt like my bones would crack.

Once Gina waved her cheery goodbye, I closed my eyes, hands draped on top of the covers, until someone showed up and had pity on me. It was my own choice when to remove these torture devices, but we all knew I should hang on as long as possible because Gina looked me in the eye every day and told me the more pain I went through now, the greater likelihood my hands would work in the future.

It was always a relief to see Bonnie walk through the door in the afternoon when the hospital routine was quiet. She usually entered tentatively, checking to see if anyone else was in the room.

When she was settled in the bedside chair, she pulled a project out of her bag. Once she made daffodils, cutting yellow paper into petals and green paper into stems and leaves. After she fastened the pieces together with glue, Bonnie assembled several flowers into a bouquet that she stuck in a plastic water bottle and placed on the bedside table.

Another day she drew a huge, red Welsh dragon and taped it to the wall beside my bed where it stayed for weeks gazing down on my struggles and small triumphs.

When Eric arrived, he found plenty to do. If the mail sat in a pile on the table, he opened each piece and read them to me. We used the alphabet device for brief conversations, but I couldn't figure out a short way to ask how he was progressing with his film projects and when he would complete his degree. Our two-way communication system was helpful for medical discussion but not much beyond that.

Stu stopped by every morning before work to give me a hug and wishes for a better day than yesterday. His longer visits came in the evenings when he read some of the cards that had arrived in the afternoon mail or recounted episodes he dealt with at work.

Sometimes after he ate a hurried, fast-food dinner, we watched videos. One of our favorites was from personal friend, Jack H, whose appearances as Director Emeritus of the Columbus Zoo on Late Night with David Letterman were hilarious, especially those episodes of hissing cockroaches crawling up Dave's arm or pythons draped over his shoulders.

Many friends had asked me over the last three months how Carole could be totally paralyzed yet her heart still beat, she could digest food, and with help from the ventilator, she could breathe.

The answer is: the nervous system is complex. Fortunately, there are two independent nervous systems at work in the body. First, the autonomic nervous system (ANS) regulates key involuntary functions like the activity of the heart, intestinal tract, glands, and the lungs. In Carole's case of Guillain-Barré Syndrome, the ANS was less affected, however, she did have irregular heart rhythms and trouble regulating her body temperature.

Second, the somatic nervous system (SNS) carries motor and sensory information to and from the central nervous system affecting the skin, sensory organs, and all skeletal muscles. This is where GBS attacked Carole the hardest.

Shortly after my brief adventure sitting on the edge of the bed, sitting in a chair became part of the daily routine. On March 29 a team of nurses, therapists, and aides moved me into a sitting position, then lifted me into a therapeutic chair. Its high back and head support were designed to cradle a patient with no body control.

Once I was propped up with pillows, everyone left the room telling me on the way out, "We'll be back in ten minutes." I couldn't imagine sitting for that long. As I gazed from wall to wall, trying to occupy my mind, the pain focused in my back, throbbing in my atrophied muscles. I managed the ten minutes that day and each subsequent day stayed in the chair a little longer, looking at my rag doll angel slumped on a nearby table, mimicking my own posture. After about a week, I could almost feel the muscles and tendons reluctantly coming back to life.

The tilt table was another device employed to get my body used to being upright. I thought of it as my own private medieval torture. The therapists slid me from the relative comfort of my bed to a gurney for the trip to the exercise room where they moved me onto the hard, brown, leather-like tilt table. Alan and Ken strapped me securely in three places with three-inch-wide straps before Alan gradually raised the head of the table to a degree that was decidedly uncomfortable.

The round, institutional clock on the wall seemed to be staring at me. I couldn't decide if it was friend or foe. When Ken told me, on the first day, I had to stay strapped to the table for ten minutes, I thought it more than unreasonable. I just looked at Ken's round red face and registered the ridiculous amount of time he expected me to hang there with nothing to do while I endured this torture. The clock stared back at me, definitely an enemy.

There was nothing to look at. Nothing to listen to. Just the clock and the pain. The black second hand swept around its circle, inching the minute hand along. I looked away from the clock and tried to think outside myself, outside the hospital walls. A glance back at the clock revealed only two minutes had passed. Eight minutes to go.

But that same clock became a friend when the hands passed the halfway mark of my assigned time because then I could focus on the countdown. I'd close my eyes or glance away, guessing how much time would run off the clock before I looked back. As I moved ever closer to the final minute, I couldn't wait to be lowered to a horizontal position to relieve the tremendous pain in my legs.

Ken walked in just as the final second ticked off, brushing back a shock of hair with his left hand. Alan lowered the table to horizontal then congratulated me on "going the distance," as the two of them lifted me onto the gurney. Once off the tilt table and back in bed, I felt almost comfortable because, although I was still in pain, it was far less than when I was on the table.

I started the tilt table on April 23, five weeks after the GBS diagnosis, and in one week I was able to tolerate a 45-degree incline. The discharge notes mention that by April 30 I was "making great strides from a rehab standpoint," referring to thirty-two days sitting in the chair, a week on the tilt table and what the physical therapists had been able to accomplish with my limbs and hands.

A major counterweight to the difficult tilt table was the comfort of a bath started on the same day. Bathing is almost an impossibility when paralyzed. In the ICU one nurse gave me a thorough sponge bath every day. This continued at ATH, but after nine weeks I longed to submerge myself in warm water.

If I thought sitting up on the side of my bed had been a huge challenge in trust, letting four nurses carry me naked into the wash room and submerge me in a tub of water was even more so. An aide untied the ugly hospital gown that always flapped open in the back and left it on the bed. Then the team of four, led by Ruthann, covered me with a light blanket and rolled the bed down the hall to the wash room, trailing my necessary medical equipment along. Once there, each of the four grabbed a corner of the sheet using it as a sling to carry me from the bed to the white enamel tub.

Steam rose in swirls above the tub which looked unusually long and very narrow. Hanging in my bed-sheet sling while an aide adjusted the water temperature, I wondered why this tub was so deep. As I watched the steam rise, I thought how good it was going to feel to be in the water, but the depth of the water frightened me. The hole in my throat where the ventilator hose was attached was a welcome funnel for water to flow into my lungs. There was no way I could control myself and slipping below the water seemed a real possibility. Finally, Phyllis turned the water off.

On Ruthann's count, "One, two, three," the nurses hefted the sheet high enough to get me over the side of the tub and then gently lowered me into the water. When my backside hit bottom, the two nurses holding my feet let go. The other nurses holding the corners of the sheet near my head assured me they would keep my head and neck above water. "Relax and enjoy your time in the water, Carole," Ruthann encouraged me. I shut my eyes and thought only of the feeling of water rippling along my body. Now I knew why the tub was narrow and deep. Total immersion felt so good and the water stayed warm.

"Can you move any parts of your body?" Ruthann asked. I found that I could move my hips slightly in a marching motion just as I had done in bed over the last week. I hadn't mentioned this to anyone because the movement was so slight I thought I must be imagining it. But with the support of the water, the movement came more easily and I rested my head against the rigid edge of the sheet, closed my eyes and nodded. The nurses, aides, and therapists all laughed and rejoiced with me.

No one hurried me through this routine. They let me relish every moment of the warm water and the freedom of being out of bed. As they dried me off, they told me I would have these baths twice a week for the remainder of my time at ATH. What a special interlude these baths were as the demands for increased activity escalated.

✻ ✻ ✻

As the myelin sheath began to regenerate around the nerves, function slowly returned. It had begun in the ICU when I was finally able to move my lips and roll my head from side to side. Now I had good control of my neck and facial muscles and could move the core of my body although not my limbs.

Time in the chair was increased every afternoon. It was still a struggle, but I could tell I was getting stronger. Soon the institutional chair that held me upright and supported my head and neck was exchanged for a regular high-backed chair. I hoped this progressive improvement would soon reach my diaphragm and allow me to resume breathing on my own. The process of weaning a patient off a ventilator was never explained, but changes in my daily routine were obviously related to this critical goal.

Each day I was asked to take a deep breath and then blow a single long breath into a clear plastic contraption. As with almost everything I did, this process was measured and recorded. The first time I was barely able to get a breath out of my lungs, but by practicing deep breathing every day, I was able to sustain longer breaths with each difficult trial.

Carole used two devices to increase her lung capacity. The most challenging required Carole to take a deep breath and blow through a hose into a plastic container with a tight-fitting plunger. At first, she could barely move the plunger. Aggravated and upset, she tried over-and-over again. It was frustrating. She hated to see Ruthann, Bonnie, or me approaching with the "breathing torture" because she knew twenty minutes of exasperation was in store. Despite Carole's frequent objections, none of us gave up because we knew she had to strengthen her chest muscles to be able to breathe on her own.

---

* Medical Appendix. Weaning from the Ventilator

The way to Dodd Hall and rehabilitation could come only when Carole was free of the ventilator.*

A bright spot amongst all this aggressive medical treatment was a letter from Katie in which she announced that not only had she received an A on her Comprehensive Final Project, Acclimatizing Snow Leopards in U.S. Zoos," but that she had been invited to present her project at two psychology conferences in the spring. What an uplifting message. Life goes on, I thought.

In the same letter, Katie wrote this about Keith.

> *"Remember the qualities I told you I would want in a guy. Well I've found a guy with all of them and more. The relationship Keith and I share is something I've never experienced before. He's someone I could spend my entire life with and never regret a moment of it. I only wish I knew what the future is going to bring."*

As Stu read this letter aloud, I smiled. My feelings when I first saw Keith in the ICU were mirrored in this letter. Katie and Keith were meant for each other.

About this time, the nursing staff introduced me to a Continuous Positive Airway Pressure circuit (CPAP). Using it, I could breathe with only slight assistance from the ventilator. At first, I wore the CPAP mask for short periods of time, but gradually increased the time as my breathing became more regular.

After my time on CPAP was significantly increased, they gave me a trach collar like the one I had used in the ICU. This device allowed me to breathe on my own through the endotracheal tube but with a flow of oxygen from the collar. There was no support from the ventilator. I built up time on both CPAP and the trach collar through April. I also wore a pulse oximeter on my finger. It measured the oxygen in my blood, an important factor in helping to determine when I would be able to go off the ventilator for good

Three months ago, Carole and I drove into a dark canyon ringed with warning signs, "GBS...proceed with caution." The winding journey through the ED and ICU was now behind us. The transfer to ATH was both a physical and psychological shift letting us know there was a way out of the abyss. Rather than the continuous slide downward, little by little we were now climbing out the far side of our own personal Grand Canyon.

Each day Carole faced and overcame new obstacles. Sometimes they were small like a stone in her path. Other times they were like a pile of boulders. Getting off the ventilator was such a challenge.

We never gave the ventilator a name but it seemed to have its own personality. An unassuming grey box, about the size of a microwave, resting on four skinny, grey legs with wheels for feet, it had dials and switches for a face. A semi-transparent tube about two inches in diameter reached out to Carole and provided her the pressurized air that was keeping her alive. We both knew Carole had to wean herself off this machine by learning to breathe again on her own.

One day, Diana told Stu and me that I was making such rapid progress, I might be able to use a device attached to the trach tube to allow me to talk.* By forcing air out of my windpipe and over the device I would be able to talk. It sounded tricky to me, but Diana forged ahead, assuring me this could be done without any danger.

"Until you build enough strength in your diaphragm to talk on your own, this device will help you speak," Diana offered.

"Just think, when you learn to use this device we will actually be able to talk to each other!" Stu encouraged me.

A few days later, Diana explained the device and technique one more time before saying,

"The first try will be hard. You may only get out a few words." She twisted the little plastic gizmo three times, then turned to me and said,

"Think about what you want to say to Stu. You're only going to be able to say a few words."

I nodded ascent as she screwed the device into place.

"Squawk, squawk."

Nothing intelligible. Another breath-whisper and very slowly I said three words I had wanted to say to Stu for months,

"Get my hairstylist!"

Poor Stu stood there staring at me. It's funny in retrospect, but at the time it was not. I had planned to tell Stu how much I loved him, but after these first three words, I had no verbal energy left. I fell back to my only other means of communication. I winked at Stu and he winked back. Our eyes met and I knew

---

* Medical Appendix. Passy-Muir Valve

the communication was complete. "I love you! Would you please contact my hair stylist?" I was disappointed in the device, and in myself. Seeing my frustration, Diana gathered her things and as she left, said,

"We'll try again in the morning when you're well rested, Carole. Please don't give up."

I did try the next day, and many more times. I got bits of sentences out but never was able to use the device the way everyone else wished I could. Maybe it was the stubborn, impatient me getting in the way of learning how to use this device. Maybe I just wanted to get off the ventilator and talk on my own.

Without warning, a critical issue surfaced – one that caught me completely off guard. Apparently, Carole needed a hairstylist in the worst way. I had no idea who her hairstylist was or whether anyone could come into the hospital to do her hair. I'd have to find another way to solve this problem.

Saturday afternoon Bill, one of Carole's weekend nurses, and I were ready. As we assembled our gear and maneuvered the bed into position, Carole gave me a look you would give your 4th grade child before he went on stage as one of the three kings in the annual Christmas pageant.

"He's so cute. He will screw up his one and only line: 'Hark. Is this where the Savior is born?' But no one will care and we will still love him." I could actually get all of that information in one glance from Carole.

As I poured warm water over her head and gently rubbed shampoo into her hair, I could see from the expression on her face that she was enjoying the relaxation. After quickly rinsing, I towel-dried her hair then grabbed the hairdryer. There! What more could a girl want? Bill and I were proud of ourselves. Of course, Carole couldn't see what her hair looked like.

A look over our shoulders at the female staff who had congregated in the entryway to the room, left me with the feeling we may have missed something. While the end result wasn't the ultimate in hairstyling, it was another step toward a normal life for Carole. And she was beginning to look like the gorgeous woman in the picture hanging at the head of her bed.

Diana was also ready to have me experiment with eating. This worried me even more than the speaking device. I was afraid of choking. I didn't know if I could make myself swallow anything. She remained optimistic and encouraging, however, assuring me we would start with very small amounts of easy-to-swallow food. Jell-O was first on the list. And despite my apprehensions, it was wonderful to feel that cool blob slide down my throat. At each meal Diana introduced new foods as she thought I could handle them. I stayed on tube feedings for now, but imagined having that tube extracted for good as I enjoyed a widening variety of soft food.

Some difficulties emerged as Diana introduced more solid foods. Swallowing crackers was particularly difficult even with liquid. Near the end of April, Dr. R ordered an X-ray of my throat to determine what was contributing to the swallowing problem.

There was a lot of chatter among nurses and therapists about the terrible radiologist we would face the day of the test. They talked openly about how gruff and unreasonable the man was and assured me that several of them would go along to ease the way.

After I swallowed a dose of barium, Diana and Gina gamely escorted me to the first floor and introduced me to the radiologist. As he grunted a response which I couldn't understand, Diana tried to explain my condition, the pain I endured, and that I was still mostly paralyzed. The radiologist said directly to me,

"Get on the X-ray table," then turned away.

Of course, it wasn't possible for me to get out of the wheelchair on my own let alone get up onto the table. Gina wheeled the chair closer to the table looking for direction from Diana. Without a word, they lifted me from both sides, grimacing as they got me on to the radiology table. It was a struggle for them, but the radiologist never turned around or offered to help.

The table was cold. The radiologist, even colder. Although he had been told I could not move on my own, he kept telling me to turn one way or the other, to move an arm or a leg. Each time one of the therapists had to assist me. The radiologist grumbled and growled as I chewed and tried to swallow various foods before each X-ray. This took far longer than the radiologist wanted to wait.

He complained and griped but never gave direction for me to do anything differently. After all, what he was checking for was why I was having such a hard time swallowing. Since there was an indication of a problem, it would have seemed reasonable for him to at least be patient if not sympathetic.

Chapter Ten

Celebrations

B y the beginning of May my recovery was progressing measurably. The tilt table was at a 50-degree angle and my time-onboard had increased beyond a half hour. While still a tedious exercise, the pain was far less. My strengthening core was evident in longer stretches sitting in the chair in the afternoon.

With a combination of CPAP and trach mask, I was off the ventilator for almost sixteen hours a day. Soon I would try to go twenty-four hours without the ventilator and accomplish breathing on my own. What scared me most about this was the psychological issue of going to sleep without the mechanical support that had kept me alive for three months.

Eating by mouth was also progressing well. The results of the X-ray showed no abnormalities, so we progressed through more complicated types of food. I was eating two regular meals a day with the help of whoever was around to feed me.

While I thought I was making great progress eating slightly mushy "real" food, the nutritionist, Dr. R, and Diana thought I needed to supplement my intake with high protein Ensure. They wanted me to drink two cans a day. This was another challenge. The amount of food I was expected to eat was insurmountable. With my stomach full after my best effort, I left much of each meal on the plate. Yet, within an hour I was presented with a can of Ensure in a plastic cup with a protruding straw. Just thinking about trying to drink it made my stomach overflow. But Ruthann forcefully insisted I drink the whole thing. With Stu's gentle encouragement, I tried to accommodate, sometimes taking the entire evening to get it down.

Taking medications by mouth was another difficult transition for me. Swallowing whole pills was impossible, but even crushed, they stuck in my throat. I coughed and gagged every time. For days, no one seemed to know how to make this easier until one night, Eric mixed the crushed pills in yoghurt. It slid right down my throat. Applesauce proved to be another helpful medium for pill-swallowing so the nurses kept both on hand to ease this daily aggravation.

Carole and I raised three wonderful children, each with distinct personalities, talents, and interests. They also share several attributes. The ones we are most proud of are their sense of integrity and devotion to each other and to us. We were reminded of this as Katie's graduation approached.

For the whole family, Katie's graduation would be special and with Carole already weaning herself from the ventilator, I wondered if I could somehow get her to Allegheny College for the ceremony. Not probable, but definitely possible. Balancing the pressures of a new job, visiting with Carole every evening, and perfecting my hair styling skills, I began to develop a plan.

I realized, no matter how rapidly she progressed in the next several weeks, she could not handle a four-hour drive each way in the family car. As I explored possibilities, a business friend of Carole's heard of my idea and contacted me.

Jerry's business is constructing and refurbishing motor homes for entertainers to travel cross-country on tour. Jerry was aware of Carole's ordeal and, like most who knew her, was a great admirer.

One night after work I stopped by Jerry's dealership where he showed me a rig with a queen-sized bed, a built-in bathtub, and a sound system powerful enough to make you think you were playing first fiddle in the Philharmonic Orchestra. Jerry offered to loan me the unit free. All I had to do was pay for the gas.

Jerry seemed to know a lot about what Carole was going through and revealed how many others were thinking of her when he said,

> *"We all know Carole's had a long struggle. There are so many of us who would like to help."*

I could barely breathe out a "Thank you."

> *"Let me know when you want the keys and forget what I said about the gas. I'll take care of that too."*

While I did not expect to leave Jerry's office with tears in my eyes, I had to gather myself before I started the car to drive to the hospital.

The possibility of Carole going to Katie's graduation suddenly seemed real. I had not shared any of these thoughts with her because she did not need the additional stress of having to meet a deadline to get off the ventilator. I did, however, share it with a few nurses and a respiratory therapist. They were guarded in their reaction. I could tell they did not want to rain on my parade, but at the same time, they did not want to be overly optimistic and raise false expectations.

I had the route figured out to avoid any two-lane roads until we got right to the campus. I called the college and talked through the logistics of parking the mobile home and escorting Carole in a wheelchair to a position where she could see the stage where Katie would receive her diploma.

One evening, Barbara, the respiratory therapist, offered to accompany us on this trip. She said she would handle the respiratory equipment and provide some limited professional care for Carole. With her assistance, I thought, this crazy idea might even get off the ground.

I made sure Barbara realized Carole need not know of my plan and promised to keep her up to date as it developed. We were still four weeks away from a "Go - No Go" decision. What I had accomplished was easy. Carole had to do the hard work of getting off the ventilator.

Katie came home from college on the 5th of May full of anticipation for graduation on the 11th. It was great to have Katie, Glen, and Eric around to talk about the upcoming graduation. But as the conversations swirled, I silently mourned that I wouldn't be there to see this important milestone in her life. The whole family would be going without me.

Through the first week of May, I breathed longer and longer on my own. The time was near to see if I could make it through the night without the ventilator. By this time, I could speak in short sentences by having someone cover the hole in my trach. Thus, I was able to talk with Stu and Bonnie about the upcoming weaning for more than a week. Stu seemed more excited than I was.

Things were beginning to fall into place. The magnificent RV was reserved and ready to go. Barbara had made her vacation arrangements. Carole was stretching her time off the ventilator to over sixteen hours at a time and I pushed, gently, for her to work harder and faster at this goal.

One Saturday morning as I walked to Carole's room, the Ward Clerk stopped me and said,

"Dr. R wants to see you in the conference room."

I walked apprehensively to the conference room and opened the door. The entire staff was assembled for their regular morning report when the night shift shares with the oncoming day shift information about the status of their patients.

"Dr. R, the Ward Clerk said you wanted to see me. Is this a good time?" He looked at me with a mixture of concern and compassion. Then right out with it, he came,

"I understand that you plan to take Mrs. Williams out of the hospital."

I had been on the vent for seventy-four days and couldn't imagine being able to breathe on my own even though I had proven I could do without the machine for sixteen hours. I thought about my lungs and the breathing process. How does the body know to breathe on its own? What if I get too tired and can't take the next breath? If I suddenly stop breathing during the night, who will know? How will I be rescued? These thoughts argued back and forth with my rational self who said,

"If you weren't ready physically, they wouldn't be proposing the overnight trial. And, certainly the nursing staff will monitor you without Stu and Bonnie having to be here."

Every day I considered whether or not I would be able to do this on my own. On the 4th I told Stu and Bonnie to plan to be with me the night of the 6th. To frustrate their efforts without having to talk with them about it, I determined to stay off the vent one night early. After they left on May 5th I told the nurses I would like to go through the night off the vent, by myself. They agreed, understanding I was going to surprise Stu and Bonnie. They got a kick out of the plan and encouraged me by saying it would not be a problem. They would be watching me.

While I had been off the ventilator since early morning, I couldn't imagine not being reconnected before I fell asleep. So, I laid there staring at the ceiling waiting for sleep to come, wondering if my internal regulator was ready for the challenge. It was later than usual when I finally fell asleep.

I woke refreshed the next morning, a big grin on my face to greet Stu when he came in around 6:30 am toting his breakfast from the hospital cafeteria.

"It's done," I said. I'm off the vent!"

What a feeling to be able to breathe on my own again. The look on Stu's face was pure joy. The ventilator that had breathed for me since February 20th was now silent. The absence of sound reminded me of the miracle of my own breathing and the fact the machine was still in the room told me if there was trouble, I could be reattached quickly, a precaution that lasted four days.

On Monday a man in a drab olive grey uniform walked up to the ventilator. He wrapped up the hoses and cords and rolled the machine out the door, never saying a word.

The day the ventilator departed, I moved the fingers on my right hand for the first time. I had been moving a few fingers on my left hand for several weeks but nothing seemed to be happening with my right hand. This was only a slight movement but definitely visible to others. Looking down my arm to my fingers, it seemed almost miraculous they could move again. I glanced up from my hand to see Gina beaming.

Even though many good things were happening in my recovery and I knew this would be a wonderful weekend for Katie, I was sad to be stuck in the hospital. The nurses were especially attentive and on Saturday put me in a wheelchair at the nurses' station where I sat chatting with whoever had time and the inclination. It took my mind off the family trip to Pennsylvania. Bonnie promised to be back on Sunday to keep me company while we thought about the rest of the family at the graduation ceremony.

"Against medical advice."

Those were the only words I could hear. Carole had spent the night off the vent. Everything was in place. Katie was graduating this weekend.

"Against medical advice." I heard the words again and snapped back to what Dr. R was saying, although I already knew.

"I am not going to allow you to do this. She is in no condition to take a lengthy trip no matter what the reason."

All heads around the table glanced down at the same time. No one wanted to look at me or at Dr. R. Apparently, the grapevine had spread the word of my elaborate plan and had embellished it a bit, as most good grapevines do. Dr. R was rightly concerned as he had received the information in its raw form, then added a few assumptions of his own.

I apologized to Dr. R and explained I was only getting prepared in case it became possible for Carole to attend the graduation. I realized he had been blind-sided and was understandably concerned that we might push the limits too far, too fast. Grudgingly, I tried to remember, we were on the same team here.

The only good news was I had not shared my grand idea with Carole. If I had, she would have been as utterly disappointed as I was. I'd have to go to graduation without her.

While Stu headed off to Katie's graduation with Eric, I never could have imagined what Bonnie was planning. She arrived at the hospital on Sunday with bags and boxes, dishes and napkins, candles and cloth.

With only a little assistance from the nurses and their agreement that she could use their break room, Bonnie set up an entire banquet: a full turkey dinner with mashed potatoes and vegetables. While that heated up, she sliced apples and spread them with melted Brie, a favorite of hers and mine. She baked rolls in a toaster oven, lit candles, and brought dinner to my bed.

The support Bonnie gave me throughout my illness was unwavering. And this special day was such a meaningful way to pass the time when both of us would rather have been in Pennsylvania. The love behind that dinner will live with me for the rest of my life.

I imagined the hill of green grass sloping down from Bentley Hall, toward the freshman dormitory where both Katie and I had spent our freshman years thirty-two years apart. That hill is dotted with huge oak and maple trees planted after the founding of the college in 1815.

Stu and I enjoyed four years of laughter and love and learning at Allegheny. We imagined Katie and Keith shared the love of the place as much as we did and that this day would be a special memory for them. It was a beautiful day and the ceremony would certainly be held outside on that gently sloping lawn under the arching majesty of those magnificent trees.

I closed my eyes and saw family and friends gathered in rows of folding wooden chairs waiting for the graduates to flow out of Bentley Hall. There would be music and speeches, joy and celebration.

As Bonnie gathered up the remains of our feast, I closed my eyes and dozed, thinking about hearing all the graduation stories on Monday. But I didn't have to wait that long.

In an unexpected surprise, Katie returned that night with Stu and Eric, and we had a wonderful time reliving the ceremony. As the conversation wound down, Bonnie handed a small package to Katie.

With Bonnie's help, I had written Katie a poem to accompany a special necklace Stu and I had designed for her. While Katie unwrapped the box, Stu quietly handed Bonnie a single gold key on a chain, a remembrance of her help in creating this memory for all of us. Bonnie stayed back, tears in her eyes, as Katie came to my bed and gave me a long hug of graduation happiness.

* * *

After the high of graduation weekend, I came back to the reality of therapy Monday morning. I could almost feel the myelin sheath growing back along the nerves and the desire to move edge back into my muscles. Four days earlier I told Stu the pain in my arms from the elbows down had increased significantly. The same was true from my hips to my feet with the greatest pain below the knees.

On May 14, almost two months after being admitted to ATH, I sat up in a regular chair for the first time. I was able to sit, propped with pillows, for forty-five minutes, yet achieving the two-hour mark required for admission to Dodd Hall still seemed a long way off so, I was surprised to learn I would be leaving ATH on May 16th. Was I really ready for this next transition?

Friday morning, I found out just how much the ATH staff cared. More than twenty people gathered in the hallway outside my room as Ruthann and Phyllis got me ready to leave.

Someone had made a large Good Luck poster filled with special messages, funny drawings, and memories of our time together. Everyone signed the card and with it gave me a list of their addresses and phone numbers.

Someone else had made a crazy bouquet of tongue depressors, rubber gloves, string, band aids, Handiwipes and Neosporin packets. Just before I was wheeled away, Diana handed me this lighthearted reminder of our two months together. I told them I'd be back for a visit, but I knew there would never be any way to tell them how very much they meant to my getting well.

I noticed through my own tears that many of them were crying.

As people gathered by the punch bowl at the nurses' station, I noticed there were several staff members in casual clothes, not their usual uniforms. I chided them about the informality but was soon corrected.

"It's my day off, but I had to come in to say goodbye to Carole," Barbara volunteered.

"Watching our favorite patient make so much progress has been an inspiration. We couldn't let her go without saying goodbye," Joel said. "I just had to be here today."

That said it all. Carole had touched these people almost as much as they had touched her. It was a graduation celebration of mixed emotions. All of them had helped Carole through an arduous physical and emotional battle. They had prepared her for the next phase of rehabilitation. While they would not see the final outcome, they had left their mark and enabled Carole to move on. In some small way, I believe Carole left her mark on them as well.

Dr. R didn't show up.

Chapter Eleven

In Over Their Heads

As the ambulance moved through Columbus' city streets, I thought about the progress I had made over the last three months. At the same time, I wondered if I was ready for the demands of rehabilitation at OSU's renowned Dodd Hall?

Breathing was comfortable now as though I had never been on a ventilator, but holding myself upright in a chair for just one hour tested my stamina. Meeting the two-hour requirement was still impossible. Would I be able to handle therapy?

It was quiet as the ambulance crew slid me quickly from the gurney into bed while a nurse named Linda asked numerous questions, recording my answers on official hospital forms.

After a check of my vital signs and a review of the medications' list, and feeding parameters forwarded by the staff at ATH, Linda had me settled in room 4149. I laid there quietly, looking at the ceiling, thinking about the challenges I was about to face.

Eric and Stu arrived with a collection of things from my room at ATH: family photos, sun catchers for the windows, books from caring friends, and posters for the ceiling. As Eric taped the large pastoral scene to the wall across from my bed, Stu unrolled a smaller Van Gogh print of sunflowers in a vase while he joked about the growing art gallery. Observing all of this activity, the little ragdoll angel rested at the foot of the bed. She appeared to wink approval of this move.

A first-year resident, Dr. A, came in to assess my condition, followed hours later by the attending physician, Dr. L.

The medical record states my condition on May 16th in stark terms. I was "maximally dependent for all aspects of mobility and active range of motion" which meant I couldn't move at all on my own.

I required maximum assistance for all activities of daily living and had only minimal movement of my head and shoulders. This meant I couldn't feed, dress, or toilet on my own.

They also noted that my upper extremity range of motion was severely limited. Even with a therapist's assistance I was unable to move my arms and fingers over a normal range of motion. My legs were worse.

Additionally, I had decreasing sensitivity in my lower legs. In other words, as they tested for feeling with a pin prick moving down each leg, they found less and less sensation. I couldn't feel a thing below the knees.

And pain was a primary concern of both the resident and the attending physician – a real change from Dr. R's attitude at ATH. Here at Dodd they knew they needed to manage the pain so I could be an active participant in therapy sessions.

That first afternoon a speech therapist came in to evaluate my language, communication, and swallowing. Progress in these areas had been faster than in any other, telling me regeneration of the myelin sheath was starting at the top of my spinal cord and moving down and out to my arms and legs. The therapist recommended no service from her department, a sign of good improvement. Her notes recorded my ability to eat puree, bread, and liquids, but that I could not feed myself.

In the afternoon, a psychology intern visited to make her evaluation. It was bleak, as well, but accurately reflected many of my concerns.

> Ms. Williams was seen for assessment of emotional and cognitive functioning. She was alert and oriented at the time of assessment. She has little functional movement aside from her head and neck. She was very tearful during this session, expressing anxiety about being in a new environment and about the expectations for performance in rehab. She displays significant adjustment issues, including concerns regarding loss of independence, as well as anxiety and mild feelings of depression regarding her illness.

Again, unlike at ATH, my anxiety and depression were acknowledged as part of the syndrome of GBS and were treated with medication and continuing visits from a staff psychologist throughout my months at Dodd Hall.*

---

* Medical Appendix. Anxiety and depression

Nursing notes from my first two days reveal many issues. I had a urinary tract infection. And, while I thought I was successfully off the ventilator, I had trouble catching my breath and complained frequently of an inability to breathe normally. Suctioning was performed but not until the afternoon of the second day was a "sticky plug" removed from my trach. After that Evelyn, the head nurse on the day shift, noted on my chart that I was relaxed and resting comfortably.

The rumor about the challenging rehab schedule was confirmed for me right away: two sessions, morning and afternoon, were required every weekday and one session on Saturday mornings. No wonder they wanted patients to be able to sit up for at least two hours at a time. Thankfully, because I was transferred on Friday, I would have just one half-day therapy session on Saturday and then Sunday to rest before beginning the grueling daily schedule the following Monday.

On Saturday morning Evelyn and two aides arrived after breakfast to get me dressed. Their shoes squeaked on the shiny tile floor as they picked up a pair of sweat pants Stu had dropped off before breakfast. The aides quickly maneuvered me into the sweat pants.

Socks and shoes followed. Braced by an aide, I was now sitting on the side of the bed looking down at the bulky athletic shoes. Ugly, but supportive I decided.

Getting a shirt over my head was an impossibility. Because my shoulders were frozen in place and my elbows at ninety-degree angles, the aides could find no way to maneuver me into a shirt. One started by putting my right hand and arm through the hole then tried to lift the shirt up over my head. My arm hadn't bent in that direction since February and it wasn't going that way today either. I tried not to scream too loudly but they got the idea this approach would not work. The second aide started differently by pulling the shirt over my head first. Then she took my left arm and tried to force it into the arm hole. No luck. I gasped with pain.

"My arms won't bend that way," I wailed, fighting back the tears.

"Well," Evelyn said with a smile, "You can't go downstairs topless."

Calmly Evelyn stretched the neck hole beyond its ability ever to recover its normal shape. After which, the aides were able to get me into the shirt. I could go to rehab that day but knew by Monday somebody would have to find a much larger shirt for me.

Now to get me out of bed and into a wheelchair. Evelyn and the aides swung into action, picking me up and placing me in the wheelchair before I had time to think about it.

As I struggled to stay upright, Evelyn attached a tray to the wheelchair arms and gently placed my hands flat on the tray. I looked down at my hands, inert on the tray, as I tipped slowly to the right. This wheelchair had a sling seat and a tubular metal frame. It would have been uncomfortable for a totally healthy person and wasn't substantial enough to support me. Evelyn saw this right away. She asked an aide to pull me up and forward while she positioned a pillow under me. Then she quickly slipped pillows on each side to hold me up. I felt much more secure and better balanced. Thoughtfully, someone stroked a brush through my hair and Evelyn announced that I was ready for rehab.

The Dodd Hall website describes their approach to rehabilitation: "We help individuals live their lives to the fullest after disabilities caused by trauma, illness, congenital deficits or disease. We combine state-of-the-art treatments with personalized care to meet each patient's unique and changing needs." I was on my way to find out how these two brief sentences are put into practice.

With a cheery, "You're good to go!" and a sharp tap on the wheelchair tray, Leon, a physical therapy aide, spun around to the back of the chair and wheeled me toward the elevator. I swayed from side to side trying to maintain an upright position to prove I was ready for this challenge although I felt far from it. Down three floors and out into the corridor we went, headed for the large physical therapy room at the end of the hall.

My eyes swept across the large gymnasium with an overabundance of equipment. The floor was lined in various places with strips of colored masking tape like markings for kindergarten relay races. Ropes hung from the ceiling and pulleys with their counterbalancing weights dangled along the wall. All around the room were wooden frames with padded blue cushions about three feet off the floor. I would spend hours on these mat tables and grow to appreciate their utility. Stationary bicycles stood in line along the windowed wall next to wooden stairs leading nowhere. Two sets of parallel bars were set at different heights. The hulk of a car loomed near the center of the room. Balls of various sizes had been rolled to the periphery and two torturous tilt tables leered at me from a corner. I looked the other way, remembering the pain of gravity's drag on the tilt table at ATH.

There were plenty of machines and gadgets, but more important were the many people with knowledge, persistence, and good cheer to encourage (and often force) all of us to fight to recover our independence.

I came in after most other patients were lined up waiting for therapy to begin. While Leon rolled me into place, I looked closely at my fellow patients, wondering what had happened to each person to bring them to Dodd. A young man with an external halo brace on his head and neck had probably been in an automobile accident. The older woman with a long white braid trailing down her back had obviously had a stroke. Her husband stood behind her wheelchair, stoic in a three-piece suit and fedora. He stared straight ahead, but occasionally stooped to whisper something to his wife. She smiled lopsidedly and nodded her agreement.

Behind this row of nineteen patients stood enthusiastic young high school students in jeans topped with red and white stripped polo shirts. Their volunteer hours would be put to good use transporting patients, assisting therapists, moving equipment to where it could be used most beneficially.

Therapists, aides, and volunteers quickly found their assigned patients and moved each of us to an appropriate work station. Stu walked in just in time to meet my physical therapist.

Richard, a tall, strong, strawberry blond introduced himself and rolled my wheelchair to one of the mat tables. In a light British accent, he explained the first thing I needed to learn: how to transfer from the wheelchair to the mat table. I understood the benefit of learning to slide on a board from one place to another but I couldn't picture how this would be possible when I couldn't hold my body up or use my hands to push or support myself. Once Richard removed the support pillows, I knew I would topple over.

Richard proceeded, though, as if there would be no problem with this exercise. He showed us a transfer board. It was thin yet strong, about three feet long and one-foot wide. Richard explained the transfer technique which involved my scooting forward in the chair, then Stu placing the board under my bottom and bridging it over to the mat table. By shifting my weight onto the board and then sliding myself along, I could maneuver onto the therapy table, Richard explained, after which he encouraged us to attempt a transfer with his assistance.

"Impossible, I thought. There is no way I can participate."

Richard realized this and said,

"Let Stu and me help you through this," as they manually slid me along the board and onto the mat table.

I sat on the edge of the table, my legs dangling to the floor. Stu held me upright while Richard considered what to do next. I was feeling frustrated and hopeless as I sat there. My head drooped. My shoulders rolled toward each other. Just as I thought "I'm not ready for this," for the third time, Richard stepped onto the table and kneeled in position while Stu dragged my inert body and positioned me comfortably in Richard's arms.

I was facing away from Richard. From this position, he explained the four muscle groups in each of my thighs, known as the quads, and asked if I thought I could move them, one at a time. I agreed to give it a try.

As Richard named each muscle and told me where it was, I tried to envision it and willed it to move. "One, two, three, four" Richard counted slowly as I tried to contract the right muscle. I couldn't feel any movement and had no feedback whether anything positive was happening or not.

We proceeded like this through all the muscles in both thighs until our therapy time was up. Stu and I gamely tried a transfer from the table back to the wheelchair and as I was wheeled off by an occupational therapist for the next phase of treatment, the consternation in Richard's face reflected my own.

Betsy, the occupational therapist, was lighthearted and upbeat as she wheeled me to another area to work on my upper body. This therapy studio had as much equipment as the physical therapy area, only smaller. Each device was designed to build strength in arms and hands. Tall, thin Betsy gave me a tour and in a gentle way pointed out various kinds of equipment we would use to bring my arms and hands back to life. I liked this charming, competent young woman.

Just as at ATH, Betsy started each session by warming my arms and hands with hot packs. She showed me a tub of hot paraffin and explained that eventually we would be able to use paraffin dips to warm and relax my hands. By dipping each hand over and over into hot wax, a thick layer formed, warming the tendons and muscles and making it easier to work the frozen joints.

Stu and I commented on the equivalent of a bicycle for the arms and hands that I would surely learn to use later when I could grip the handles. Another device of wood, ropes, and pulleys would stretch my arm muscles, loosen up the shoulder joints and begin to rebuild lost muscle tissue.

Seeing a room of computers, I wondered aloud,

"Do you think I'll ever be able to keyboard again? I'll need to when I return to work."

Betsy in her quiet way assured me, "Yes, of course you will."

"I guess we won't start that today," I joked.

Betsy set her shoulder length light brown hair swirling as she twirled away laughing and said,

"Not today, but sooner than you might think."

This first day we didn't do any therapy. Certainly, Betsy observed during this orientation session that I was minimally functional. I wondered if she was as perplexed as Richard seemed to be despite her upbeat attitude.

The following Monday Betsy did a full occupational therapy evaluation, revealing high cognitive functioning but performance activity registering as "Total Assistance" needed in every functional area. As Betsy asked questions and requested me to attempt various movements, I knew the report would be bleak. Indeed, the report drew a dismal picture of the daunting challenge Betsy and I would face in the days and weeks ahead.

This short Saturday morning introduction to physical and occupational therapy was finally over. Reinforced in my view that it was a blessing to have arrived on a Friday, I returned to my room and gratefully eased back into bed.

By Monday morning, routine blood work drawn on admission showed a minor urinary tract infection. The resident, Dr. A, took immediate action and put me on a course of antibiotics that would throw my schedule and the initiation of rehabilitation into chaos.

A side effect of this treatment is severe diarrhea which affected me mentally and emotionally as well as hampering my first efforts at the rigors of rehab. Of necessity, I had to wear diapers for eighteen days. This was particularly disturbing in therapy where I was with many other patients and therapists. It was difficult enough to concentrate on the demands of therapy without having to worry if I was going to embarrass myself.

If the treatment for the urinary tract infection had been necessary, I could have put up with it for eighteen days with better humor, but it turned out the treatment was not necessary at all.

One morning a few days after I had been put on antibiotics, Stu overheard Dr. L, talking with a group of residents on rounds. My assigned resident explained about the urinary tract infection he had detected and the course of treatment he had initiated. The attending physician, in a controlled burn, explained to the resident that the infection was minor and could have been treated with cranberry juice.

How could Dr. A not understand the embarrassing consequences of his decision? The reason I was at Dodd Hall was for aggressive rehabilitation. I was not going to be excused from therapy because of diarrhea. Anything that slowed my progress was a problem for me. On top of which, insurance coverage for rehabilitation was severely time-limited. I needed every hour of every day to be productive.

The consequences of having diarrhea had me longing for a trip to the washroom where, as at ATH, I might relax in a tub of hot water. This solution for cleanliness wasn't offered, but one afternoon tall, bold Kaila showed up in her purple aide's uniform to tell me it was time for a shower. Enthusiastically, she approached the bed and said,

"Let's get ready to go."

"How will I shower when I can't stand up or even sit on my own?" I wondered aloud.

"Not a problem," Kaila remarked as she took off my hospital gown and covered me with a sheet.

With help from Evelyn and a second aide, I was moved to a plastic-covered gurney that Kaila deftly maneuvered into the hall. I turned my head in her direction to engage in conversation as we seemed to race toward the shower room. Kaila's wiry red hair was a profusion of joyous color, contrasting starkly with her purple uniform.

"This is going to be like going through a carwash," Kaila explained with a cheery laugh.

And, indeed it was. Once the gurney was rolled into position, Kaila turned on the water full blast and directed the spray over my body. Startled, I gasped with surprise and squeezed my eyes tightly shut as the spray pelted my body. After a thorough lathering with soap, Kaila shot the penetrating spray over every part of my body again. As she finished with one side, she rolled me to the other, spraying all the while.

Not exactly like the slow-paced, calm routine at ATH where I was encouraged to enjoy a soak in the tub. This was a super-efficient whizzbang cascade of water. As Kaila dried me off, I felt happy to be clean, but I certainly wasn't relaxed.

My first full week of therapy was discouraging. Richard asked every day if I could help him with a transfer from the wheelchair to the therapy table? No, I hadn't gained any function since the previous Saturday. And, although Richard persisted with the thigh flexing exercise, I still couldn't do that either. By Friday we hadn't made any progress at all. A precious week wasted.

Occupational therapy was somewhat better because Betsy could work my hands and arms without needing my assistance. She worked each joint trying to loosen up the tendons and stimulate the muscles. But if there was any improvement in function, I couldn't notice it and Betsy didn't comment.

Realization of how far Carole had come was made crystal clear when Dr. H, Dean of the Medical School, stopped by for a visit the Monday after Carole's transfer to Dodd Hall. We knew each other from my days at Children's Hospital, and Carole had done some public relations work for the Dean the year before.

After Dr. H talked amiably with Carole for a few minutes, I walked with her to the main lobby. We were exchanging thoughts about developments at the Medical School when our conversation circled back to Carole.

"Carole really looks fine, Stu," the Dean offered.

"I'm looking for more substantial signs of progress," I worried, "It's been three months already and she can barely move on her own."

"It will take a while longer, but with her determination and the care here at Dodd, I have no doubt that she will make a full recovery. She is well past the time when she could have died."

"She could have died?" my mind shrieked silently. "When was that?!"

"Take care. I'll stay in touch," Dr. H finished as she turned and strode off to her next appointment.

I could take you to the spot in the Dodd Hall lobby when Dr. H said, "when she could have died." No one told me she could have died. I looked back through all those days and nights and realized I had never completely understood what ALL the possibilities were. It never entered my mind that Carole would do anything but get better, return home and we would get on with our lives.

Chapter Twelve

Aggressive Therapy

Early in the week Dr. M, who I hadn't seen since leaving the ICU in mid-March came in to test my reflexes. Then he asked me to grab his fingers and squeeze – the strength test. This was still impossible as I couldn't lift my arms nor move my hands to grasp his fingers. He found I had almost no reflexes, and my strength was nil.

Though Dr. M maintained a neutral expression, I found out later from my medical record that he was extremely worried about my lack of progress.* Keeping his concerns to himself, he ordered intravenous immunoglobulin (IVIg), a continuation of what he had prescribed when I was in the ICU and which had not been administered during my two months at ATH.

Later, after morning therapy, Stu and Bonnie surprised me with a pass to leave the hospital. Propped in a wheelchair, pillows stuffed sides and back and a blanket wrapped around me, I felt like a cocooned insect ready to face the cool spring wind.

Stu pushed while Bonnie, walking alongside, chatted about the progress we were making, as we traveled the short distance to Rhodes Hall, then up to the ICU on the tenth floor.

I was excited to talk with the fabulous nurses who cared for me in those critical early days in the hospital. I wanted to thank them for getting me through that phase of my illness and to show them the progress I had made since leaving them nine weeks earlier.

As we approached the nurses' station, recognition lit the faces of Jane and Sally who called others on the floor to come and say hello.

---

* Medical Appendix. Axonal Damage.

Amid congratulations on my progress, I tried to take in the physical environment in the ICU. It wasn't anything like what I remembered. The rooms were much smaller. And, while there was a lot of hustle bustle, the general atmosphere was quiet. I had thought of the ICU as a noisy place.

A nurse's question about Dodd Hall brought me out of my reverie and I answered with an observation about the progress I was making. They may have wondered why I was still unable to walk or move my arms and hands, but they didn't reveal their inner thoughts.

All too soon, Stu wheeled me toward the elevator and announced another surprise. A picnic in a nearby park. It was an especially thoughtful effort to get me away from the hospital for some normal activity. Except they had no idea how painful this excursion was becoming. I kept telling myself to relax, to push the pain to the back of my mind, and to concentrate on staying in a sitting position.

The non-hospital food was delicious, probably even more so because of the beautiful spring-time view of the river winding its way through campus and south to the city's center. I took the small bites Stu spooned into my mouth and chewed them carefully as Diana had taught me to do. But suddenly manicotti stuck in my throat. Coughing and gagging, I tried to clear my throat as Bonnie and Stu hurried to help me keep breathing.

This is a common problem for people recently off a ventilator, but none of us was prepared for a choking episode out here by the river. Stu, recalling past experiences dealing with my medical emergencies, calmed me down and helped clear the blockage. While I waited for my heartbeat to return to normal, Stu and Bonnie packed up the remnants of our picnic and soon we were headed back to the hospital.

The speech therapist worked with me over the next few weeks to teach me how to avoid choking, obviously a result of the episode at the river. She instructed me to lower my chin toward my chest and then swallow. This did help but I pondered whether I was going to have to use this technique for the rest of my life or if I would eventually recover a proper swallowing reflex.

Sunday was a true day of rest after a very exciting Saturday. Stu noted on the bedside calendar my physical status on May 25th in layman's terms. In my trunk from mid-chest up I was pain free. There was tingling in my arms from elbows to wrists and in my legs from waist to knees. More of my fingers were moving slightly. These seemed like hopeful signs.

Pain was intense in my hands and from the knees down through my feet. We guessed this was progress even though I had almost no movement in my limbs.

We also guessed these new feelings in my arms, hands, and legs might be a result of the IVIg infusion.

By Monday a routine was developing just as it had at ATH and in the ICU before that. I was greeted by up-at-dawn Stu who had already fed and walked the dogs and driven to the hospital to feed me breakfast before going to work. I smiled inside at how wonderfully caring he is, and outside just to let him know how much I loved him.

* * *

After therapy on my second Friday at Dodd Hall, a bundle of energy bounced into my room and introduced herself to me and Eric. Petra was a physical therapist I had seen treating other patients while I worked with Richard. She was full of personality and determination.

Petra chatted amiably, exuding confidence and a focused energy, another of the many people who wanted to learn more about my complicated case. But in every other respect she was different. Petra was determined to find out what could be done to motivate my own drive to get well.

Light brown hair framed her face and I noticed how fit and trim she was as her penetrating gaze captured my full attention. Petra expressed the hope I wanted to feel inside: that I could achieve a total recovery. She was the first physical therapist who spoke directly to me with a sense of enthusiasm for a challenge we could face together; the first to ask what I was feeling and what I wanted to accomplish in my own therapy. Wow! I finally felt there was real hope.

"I'm the PT scheduled to be here over Memorial Day weekend," Petra offered.

"If it's OK with you, I'd like to stop by to work with you."

"Oh, that would be great," I joyfully replied, thinking I might be able to make some real progress with someone who was so enthusiastic about the possibilities.

With the promise of another visit on Saturday, Petra took what she had learned and skipped out of the room. Eric turned his head to look at me. Eyebrows raised, he asked,

"Did she really just skip away?" I smiled.

"Yes, I think she did."

On Saturday Petra tested my physical capabilities as well as my determination. Had Richard mentioned to Petra that I didn't seem interested in therapy or that I didn't try hard enough?

Petra asked if I would like to sit up on the side of the bed. Thinking back to ATH and the fear of my first experience sitting up, I was hesitant to try this with just one person helping, especially someone so small. Would she be able to support me? While I expressed this concern, Petra just kept encouraging me to an upright position and soon she had adeptly maneuvered me to the edge of the bed with my feet dangling toward the floor. I felt comfortable and not at all afraid.

Petra had a way about her that gave me confidence and her strength surprised me. She knew just where to hold on and how to guide me. She was so joyous about this accomplishment, she made me happy I could do something on my own. All 5 feet, 98 pounds of her didn't seem enough to steady me, but it wasn't a problem for Petra. Her boundless energy was buoyed by a take-charge personality and iron-willed determination.

With this one achievement between us, she called a happy farewell and was off to check on other patients. For the first time in three months I had immeasurable hope.

❊ ❊ ❊

It was the perfect time for an upbeat day. Sunday was my 54th birthday and I finally felt I might be able to make a full recovery. My mother and sister Barbara drove from Pittsburgh for a small birthday celebration. I felt almost normal as we sat in the patient lounge and chatted about my progress and what was going on with Barbara's two children back home. My mother was quiet and I wondered what fears she held inside about my future.

Mom sent me cards every week, some with long notes of encouragement and others with just a few words of love and hope. Each card was the same: a fuzzy brown, cartoonish bear sitting on a mound of grass and flowers, head on his right-hand gazing into the distance. Perhaps this is how she felt: pensive and uncertain.

Because of the holiday, there was no therapy on Monday so on Tuesday, my second full week of therapy at Dodd Hall began. Richard greeted Petra when she entered the therapy room.

"So, Petra, did you have a nice weekend?"

"I did. I had a great time with Carole. And I've been thinking about her case. Let me know if you would like some help," Petra offered, being considerate of Richard's position as my therapist.

"Let's see how things go," Richard said as he contemplated Petra's offer, perhaps a godsend to Richard who was obviously trying to help me, but was pessimistic about the eventual outcome.

During my first week at Dodd, Richard had asked Stu and me,

"What are your goals for your time at Dodd Hall?"

Stu responded, "Our goal is to have Carole walk out of the hospital at discharge."

"I'm sorry, Mr. Williams," said an astonished Richard,

"You and Mrs. Williams need to set more realistic goals."

Contrasting his attitude with Petra's, I recognized how each made me feel inside. Richard made me feel discouraged and hopeless. With Petra's approach, I felt hopeful. I just knew I could get better and after only two encounters, I had confidence she would find the best ways to help me reach my goals. When Stu and I told her one of our goals was for me to walk out of this hospital, she said she would help us make that happen. What a difference.

With Richard's agreement, Petra was soon in charge of my case and worked for the rest of my stay at Dodd Hall with doctors, nurses, and therapists to start me on an aggressive rehabilitation plan. I don't know how much she knew about Guillain-Barré Syndrome when I showed up at Dodd Hall, but by the time she took my case, she knew more than anyone else about how she would motivate me to succeed.

I didn't realize it at the time but over the long weekend, Petra conceived a full plan for my rehabilitation. As she tells it now, years later, she couldn't sleep on Friday night just thinking of the challenges I posed. Then on Saturday she dreamed about me and how to make my therapy work.

※ ※ ※

On Tuesday June 3, Betsy started the promised procedure of waxing my hands. After patiently dipping each hand in liquid wax over and over, she wrapped them tightly in yards of white bandages. The warmth soothed the muscles, tendons and bones in my hands, preparing them for Betsy's therapies.

After twenty minutes of soothing warmth, Betsy unwrapped one hand and worked the wrist and finger joints just as Gina had done at ATH. They hurt less than they had a month earlier, but the pain was still intense. So, as Betsy worked on one hand, I propped the other on the wheelchair tray and watched other patients go through their exercises, trying to remove myself from the pain.

The older woman with the long white braid was making progress recovering from her stroke. With encouragement from her husband and therapist, she could now walk fifteen feet toward the middle of the physical therapy room. As they both delighted in her achievements, I could see she would be leaving for home very soon.

The going was slower for the young man with the head injury, but he was there every day just like the rest of us, working on what was possible and hoping for the impossible. Everyone wanted to walk out of Dodd Hall and return to a normal life. For some this would be possible. Others would have to learn to cope with limitations of varying degrees. I wondered what my fate would be.

Two other areas of my body were as difficult to work on as my hands. My elbows, still frozen at ninety-degree angles, needed to be stretched back to normal range. This was extremely painful, but I could see the need for aggressive therapy here.

From being in bed so long, my shoulders were rounded and the tendons and muscles in the front of my chest were contracted, pulling my shoulders toward each other. Betsy devoted a portion of each therapy session to stretch those contracted muscles using a pulley system hanging on the wall and her own forceful maneuvers. Both shoulder blades and elbows seemed unyielding.

On Wednesday Petra asked a startling question,

"Would you like to go swimming?"

"Oh, I don't think I can do that."

"Sure, you can. A workout in the therapy pool will be soothing and let you practice standing upright. The water will support you."

"What if I fall? I'll drown."

"I'll be with you every minute. I won't let you fall."

There was no talking her out of it, so on Friday Eric and Petra got me ready for a trip to the pool. Evelyn dressed me in a swimsuit, much easier to get into than a T-shirt, then wrapped me in a blue and white striped beach towel Eric had bought for the occasion. He hung a second red and white striped one over his shoulders while we waited for Tony to appear.

Tall and good looking, Tony swept into the room, made a quick turn behind the wheelchair and boomed, "Let's get going!" Off we went, a short parade of four headed for the pool.

If I had been petrified of sitting up for the first time, going into water was twice as terrifying. One miscalculation by the person holding on to me and I would be under water with no way of saving myself. I kept thinking of Petra slipping and letting go of me or that I would be too heavy for her and she would lose her grip.

Tony and his sidekick, Leon, easily lifted me out of the chair and carried me to the pool where they deftly sat me on the edge with my feet dangling into the water. Petra, waiting there, guided me gently off the ledge to a standing position in the shallow end of the pool.

"Don't worry," Petra said, "I've got you."

"I'm here, too," Tony offered as he slipped into the water and made his way to my side. Eric stood by the wheelchair, a look of awe on his face.

Petra held both my hands as we walked down a slope until the water was chest high. She supported me easily, letting me walk the width of the pool on my own. While she kept me from falling, I moved my legs in a walking motion. Just like the time she helped me sit up in bed, I felt her encouragement and her joy in my accomplishment. She knew just how to take me at my current level of possibility and move me slightly beyond it. Progress every time we were together. I found this an amazingly inspiring approach. No task seemed too difficult and she was pushing me to greater achievements every day.

※ ※ ※

On Saturday, June 7, I spent twenty minutes on the tilt table. It is difficult to explain how tiring and painful this is, but if I was to walk again, I had to prepare my entire body for the experience.

Once the straps were secure, Jeff tilted the table to the prescribed incline of fifty-five degrees, higher than my last effort at ATH. He fixed the table in place and checked the clock.

"The goal today is twenty minutes," Jeff announced as he turned and walked away. No conversation, just a rigid, difficult goal.

"But this is a steeper angle than I'm used to."

"Time to get used to a bigger angle," he threw over his shoulder in a friendly way, "You can do it. It's only twenty minutes."

After five minutes, I thought I couldn't stand it any longer. My legs throbbed. My back ached. This was so unlike my time in the pool where my body felt weightless. Here on the tilt table, I felt hundreds of pounds of pressure pushing from my head down through my feet. Just as at ATH, there was nothing to look at but the clock. I closed my eyes, trying to think of pleasant places, but the pain was too much to let my mind escape.

Finally, right at the stroke of twenty minutes, Jeff walked through the door and lowered the table. As he lifted me into a wheelchair for the ride back to my room, he explained,

"You're going to be here every day for time on the tilt table."

"Really? Every day!" I couldn't believe it.

"Yes," he said, "You're really making progress now. We'll increase the time at fifty-five degrees and then increase the angle when you're ready."

Thankfully it was Saturday again. When I finished the half day of therapy and time on the tilt table, Stu – day pass in hand – took me to see our horses. The mare, Beauty Straw, had given birth to a filly while I was at ATH. Now spunky Beauty Star ran around her mother in the paddock. I sat in the car, my ankles throbbing from the extended stay on the tilt table, and enjoyed the pastoral setting, the sunshine, and the smell of manure.

Chapter Thirteen

Day Tripping

*T*he sun set as I drove in the driveway and opened the door for Max and Smokey who greeted me with wagging tails and cold noses. The three of us took a long, meandering walk in the woods and I quietly thought how far Carole had come since February. There was a lot to worry about, but there was also a lot to be grateful for.

At the top of the list was Petra who I had met only briefly Memorial Day weekend, but had heard much about from Carole. In just a couple of minutes this morning, I could tell why Carole was so uplifted by this new addition to her team. Petra's enthusiasm was as contagious as it was genuine. Carole's case was complex and challenging. Rather than intimidate Petra, it seemed to challenge her to learn as much as she could about GBS and how to move Carole toward recovery.

During therapy the expression on Carole face was a new one. It was one of confidence. I could see in her eyes a new level of determination that had not been there for months.

I found myself responding to therapy and the advances I was making with joy and excitement and yet when I returned to my room, doubts bedeviled my mind. I cried frequently and yet didn't want to disappoint Stu who was always encouraging me to look at the bright side and to have hope for the best possible outcome.

It seemed ungrateful to complain about how long my recovery was taking. Bonnie still visited on her days off. Eric still came to the hospital every day. And when Glen was not working, he showed up with a joke, a funny story, or just quiet reassurance. Stu was letting more friends visit too, so there was plenty of distraction. But my displays of emotion were frequent and eventually brought Pat, the psychology intern, to visit every day after therapy.

I didn't think I needed a psychologist, but Pat was a good listener and pulled thoughts out of me that I wasn't sharing with anyone else. She got me to express my frustrations and my fears. She let me cry and provided realistic suggestions to change what I didn't like and accept, for now, what I couldn't change. I don't know if my family realized how stressful this recovery was or whether Pat explained that I needed medication for my anxiety, but they never spoke of it.

The next two weeks flew by with visible progress every day. On June 8th Stu and Eric prepared me for my first home visit. After the early morning routine of bathing, dressing, and eating breakfast, they helped me into my wheelchair and took me to the car. I had gained enough strength to assist Eric and Stu as they moved me through a board transfer, but they still had to tug and pull me from the wheelchair to the car seat. We congratulated ourselves on our growing proficiency as Stu started the car.

As we rounded the last bend, Bonnie and the dogs bounded down the driveway amidst a profusion of yellow ribbons tied on the trees lining the driveway. What a welcome. I cried for joy at being back home and for sadness that I wouldn't be able to walk up to the front door.

As Eric wheeled me up a ramp from the garage into the tiled hallway leading to the kitchen, I faced more mixed emotions. When we had designed and built this house five years before, a friend had suggested we make it wheelchair accessible since we planned to retire here. I understood, theoretically, why that might be a prudent idea, especially because it was suggested by a business colleague who, himself used a wheelchair, but dismissed the suggestion because I never thought either one of us would have to use one.

Knowing Stu wanted me to enjoy the day, I tried to push all these negative thoughts to the back of my mind. We relaxed the day away trying to get used to the idea that, fairly soon I would have to function in a normal, everyday environment without the support of all the people who had been helping me cope. How would I maneuver in the kitchen? I couldn't reach the counters from the wheelchair and I certainly wouldn't be able to stand. Some of my fingers moved slightly, but my hands were essentially useless. I would never be able to cook for myself or anyone else.

Laundry might be doable once my hands and arms regained more movement. At least I might be able to load the washer and dryer from the wheelchair. All these thoughts depressed me as I tried to appear happy that I was finally able to make a trip home.

Stu placed me on the sofa where I could look out the window into the forest. The tops of the trees rooted in the ravine were swaying in a light breeze. We chatted for a while. I slept and then struggled with the convenience of a portable toilet, necessary because my knees wouldn't bend enough for me to get down to a regular one.

It was humiliating to have my husband and children move me from the wheelchair to the portable toilet and back again. They had to get me in and out of my clothes as well as move my body. I had become so used to having nurses handle all my personal needs, but somehow this was entirely different. But there was no alternative. I smiled and thanked and cringed all at the same time.

By the end of that long and exhausting day I was ready to return to the hospital where nurses and therapists gave me a sense of security I didn't feel in my own home. I sighed thankfully as they placed me back in my hospital bed and wondered when they planned to send me home for good. I wasn't nearly ready.

✳ ✳ ✳

The pace of physical therapy picked up considerably under Petra's guidance. On Monday both Stu and Eric were out of town so I faced my routine without family support. Following therapy and lunch, I was moved to the tilt table inclined to seventy degrees. I tolerated that angle for twenty minutes, remarkable progress since last Saturday.

In the afternoon, my eight-year old granddaughter, Alexandra, visited. It must have been rather frightening for her to see me in the hospital looking so different from the last time we were together in the winter. No more joking, laughing grandmother able to go on walks or play games. This grandmother was stuck in bed and looked lots older than Alex probably remembered. Eric told me that he and Alex's mother had prepared her to see a sick grandma, but Alex was unusually quiet and stayed a distance from the bed until we got to talking a little bit and she saw that no matter how I looked or where I was, I was still her grandma.

Soon Alex was talking and smiling her broad smile with typical eight-year-old gaps between her permanent and baby teeth. It was such a joy to have her visit. She reminded me why I needed to work even harder at therapy, so I could actively share the special times of her growing up.

The next day I found I could lift both knees off the bed at the same time and fold myself into a ball. Though I wobbled from side to side, I kept my balance and didn't fall over. I was gaining trunk strength every day. More tilt table that day and the next when I reached 80 degrees for fifteen minutes. We also practiced various kinds of transfers with Eric assisting. This was getting much easier which told me many muscles were getting stronger. I could be part of the process now rather than just letting other people maneuver me from place to place.

On Wednesday, with Petra's encouragement, we set a goal that I would stand up on Friday. Wow! Would I be able to do that?

It was exciting and frightening at the same time. After transferring from the wheelchair to the matt table, Petra explained what I needed to do to get myself to a standing position. As always, she briskly assured me I would be successful at this next challenge. She was cheerful yet intense in getting me ready. She wrapped my knees in strong braces and set a special, tall walker near me so I would have something to lean on once I was standing.

With Petra helping physically and encouraging verbally, I hesitantly pulled myself up to a standing position. It took all my concentration and strength.

"Grab the walker here. Lean forward now. Try to use your legs to lift yourself up," Petra guided.

"Where's the best place to grab on this walker once I'm standing?" I asked, not knowing how this was supposed to work with a contraption that came almost to my armpits.

"Just hold on to each side, right there on the top."

"Okay, got it."

Once up, it was difficult to maintain the position for more than a few minutes, but I stood as long as I could, swaying from side to side, then collapsed slowly back onto the matt table, realizing the benefit of every day on the tilt table. Just a short time standing, but this was a huge achievement. For the first time, I had real hope of walking again. Petra encouraged me to stand again and together we made it up and down a couple of more times that day.

Progress was coming in my arms and hands, too. The same day I stood up in the physical therapy room, I touched my chin with my right thumb while working with Betsy. With this range of motion, she said, I would be feeding myself soon.

Another weekend had arrived and we took advantage of good weather and two day passes to get out both Saturday and Sunday. It was still a trial to get into the wheelchair, out of the hospital, and into the car, but Stu and I were both comfortable now using the transfer board on our own.

We stopped to pick up some lunch, then drove to a spot on the river where we watched ducks and geese swimming in the shallows. I found myself wanting to stay longer rather than yearning to return to the hospital as I had done just last weekend.

The day passes required that I return to the hospital by 4:00 pm and this time we just made it back. We knew we would be getting out again on Sunday so parted with promises of a great time at home the next day. It turned out to be another relaxing day. Glen, Eric, Stu, and I watched the U.S. Open on TV most of the afternoon. And as we celebrated Father's Day over dinner, we thought of Katie traveling with friends in Europe.

The second week of accelerated progress was even better than the first. I walked in the shallow end of the pool using a walker. And the tilt table had been increased to eighty degrees for thirty minutes. Each day I practiced standing with the tall walker, my elbows resting on the high platform, and by Monday Petra removed the knee braces and let me try it without that artificial support.

I walked a few steps each day that week, increasing my endurance and rebuilding my leg muscles. Looking down, I focused all my attention on my legs, carefully putting one foot in front of the other. Each foot felt like a lead weight, and I thought I might look a bit like Frankenstein listing from side to side as I pushed the giant walker in front of me.

By the end of the second week of major progress I could touch the index fingers of both hands to the corresponding thumbs. After therapy when I was in bed by myself, I practiced this exercise over and over again, mentally reaching for the day I would finally hold a fork and feed myself.

The increased exercise brought on a new kind of pain, but this was one I was glad to have. My muscles were sore from the workout they were getting every day and while it was bothersome, I knew it reflected my increasingly rapid recovery. It reminded me of the pain I had after a good workout at the Capital Club or a three-mile run along the Olentangy River.

After this time of rapid progress, things settled back to a slower pace as if my body needed to adjust to the dramatic changes of these two exhilarating weeks. And we all rejoiced in my lengthening attention span and joy interacting with visitors.

In the middle of the week Stu's younger brother Don, wife Molly, and their youngest daughter Betsy came from Pittsburgh for a visit. Now that I could sit in the visitors' lounge, it was easier to have people come to Dodd Hall where we could talk about the progress I was making and about the future when I would be back to normal and our families could do things together again.

Steve, the OSU professor, still brought joy to my heart when I heard his hearty laugh out in the hall. He often arrived at lunchtime when he readily pitched in to feed me. Pulling a chair up to my bed, he grabbed a spoon and tackled the tray of food, always talking enthusiastically about OSU sports, his wife's aggressive tennis game, or the well-wishes of mutual friends.

Letters, cards, and flowers continued to come in from people in Columbus and around the country. Now when the mail came, Eric or Bonnie opened them and handed each one to me to read. It was so nice to be a participant in sorting through the mail.

One treasured communication arrived in a small package. It was a video tape of a raft trip down the Colorado River in the Grand Canyon. Longtime friends, Doug and Karen, had planned this trip with us the year before. When we couldn't go in May, they went on their way, camera in hand, recording the entire trip – from the helicopter ride into the Canyon, through the rapids and out into Lake Powell – to give us a sense of that fabulous trip.

I spent the afternoon listening to Karen's voice thrill at the adventure and wishing we had been along. It was almost as good as being there to hear Karen describe the chill of cold water bubbling around her head when she jumped in to ride the current out into Lake Powell. This tape and the accompanying photos were another inspiration: I wanted to get all my function back so I could enjoy adventures again with family and friends.

Now that my attention span was longer, Eric brought in several games to entertain me. One was a complicated London mystery format with maps and complicated instruction booklets. Very soon we found my attention span wasn't long enough yet for Sherlock Holmes mysteries, so we settled on Yahtzee, tucking away the more complicated game for later.

I had also been thinking more about Katie who was due back from Europe this week. Stu had secured a pass to get us out of the hospital at night, an unusual breach of protocol. But her plane was to arrive at 8:05 pm so we felt sure we could be back by 9:30 pm at the latest. That morning in therapy I walked two hundred feet from the physical therapy room to the elevator, a great accomplishment I couldn't wait to share with Katie.

We joined the parents and siblings of Katie's best friend, Tamara, and the young man they were traveling with at the airport around 7:30 pm. I, of course, was in the wheelchair. Waiting until 8:00 pm was a breeze. I could now handle that much time in the wheelchair without any pain. I chatted with the group of people waiting together and occasionally glanced out the window to see if the plane had landed.

Time dragged on past the scheduled arrival time. Then a delay was posted. What a disappointment. Stu took the opportunity to roll me around the airport. When we got back to the gate, another delay had been posted.

As the clock hands moved toward 10:00 pm, I not only felt the pain of a long day in therapy and the regular, never ending pain of GBS, but I was exhausted. I tried to move around in the wheelchair but couldn't find a comfortable position. I wondered if Stu should take me back to the hospital, but he assured me the nurses would be okay with my being late. So, we waited and waited.

When I felt like I couldn't sit up any longer, the plane finally arrived. Katie, Tamara, and Mike came into sight carrying bursting backpacks, the last people off the plane. We exchanged greetings and hugs all around as Stu collected Katie's luggage and got us moving toward the car, knowing I was at the far end of my ability to cope.

Chapter Fourteen

Fighting to Get Out

During a routine physical exam, Dr. A, the resident, detected an infection around the toenail on my right big toe. He told me,

"Carole, you need laser surgery to clean out the infection in your toe."

"That's going to stop my physical therapy. I'm just beginning to walk."

"Well, we have to operate. You have an infection."

"Please don't do this," I begged.

Dr. A's insistence ran headlong into my determination not to have the surgery now.

"I've had these infections before. A simple cleaning and antibiotics always works to clear it up. Can't we try that?"

"Surgery is necessary, Carole."

Then Katie joined the battle of the toe. Eric was already on my side and had been trying to reason with the resident. Now it was three against one and we had a showdown in the physical therapy room. I found myself sitting quietly, letting my son and daughter argue with the physician. Usually, I would have been in the forefront arguing my own case, but this time it was comforting to have two competent adults put the case out there for me.

That day I walked five hundred feet with a walker. Stu gave me a big hug before I sat down in the wheelchair. No, toe surgery was not going to stop the progress I was making. For the next three days, I practiced walking with water support in the pool and with the walker in the physical therapy room. Then it was home for the weekend where I walked in the driveway, visited with neighbors, and enjoyed Katie's travel stories and Glen and Eric's hijinks. Max and Smokey curled up next to me whenever I rested on the couch.

It was the last Monday in June. I'd been at Dodd Hall for more than six weeks and was making the kind of progress my neurologist, had been expecting for months. My spirits were high as I hoped for more improvement every day. And then I was told I would be going for toe surgery that morning instead of going to the therapy room. I was devastated. And I was mad. Dr. A had prevailed on the attending physician and the decision had been made that this surgery was absolutely necessary.

The procedure was simple. I was back in my room in less than an hour with a huge bandage around my toe and no therapy scheduled for that day. Immediately I asked Dr. A,

"How am I going to be able to continue with my therapy tomorrow?"

"Have Stu cut a hole in your shoe so the toe won't be pinched," was his helpful suggestion.

This reminded me of the diarrhea episode when the same Dr. A threw a roadblock in the way of physical therapy. Of course, it was his job to keep me healthy, but every additional burden ambushed the limited time I had left at Dodd Hall.

Stu, cheerful and upbeat as always, said, "It will be easy to modify your shoe." He found a scissors and cut a large hole in the top of the shoe to accommodate the injured toe and its voluminous bandage. Dr. A looked on approvingly, then advised,

"Your left big toe looks as if it might need surgery, too."

I rebelled internally at this news without saying a word to Dr. A.

"Absolutely not," I wailed to Stu when we reached the privacy of my room.

"They will have to do something else with this toe. I will not have surgery on both feet just when I'm beginning to walk."

Because this toe was not yet infected, just red, Dr. A eventually agreed to use a topical antiseptic to try to control the problem. Thankfully, this was good enough and that toe never needed surgery.

The toe surgery did little to slow the demands for continual improvement that met me every morning in the gym. The therapists seemed to be trying to get as much instruction into my head and training into my recovering body as fast as they could. Increasing discussion of the inevitability of the end of medical benefits for inpatient therapy suggested I would soon be sent home to finish recovering on my own.

A week or so before the toe surgery, Betsy had introduced me to a "dressing stick." It was about a yard-long with a grasping mechanism on the end. By squeezing a lever on the top end of the stick, I was, theoretically, supposed to grab a piece of clothing with the pincers and maneuver it to a position where I could grab it with my hands. Trying to put shorts on in this manner illustrated the complexity and frustration of using a dressing stick.

At first, I looked like a toddler with a pull toy. My crude grasp allowed me to maneuver the stick toward the shorts, but my fine motor coordination wasn't good enough to press the lever and keep the stick near enough to the shorts to grasp them. Betsy encouraged me to try again and when I couldn't work the stick properly, she helped me get dressed, assuring me we would try again the next day.

After several days of frustration, I was able to dangle the shorts from the stick and maneuver them toward my legs. Sitting on the edge of the bed with my feet hanging over the edge, I was supposed to hit both leg holes with the correct feet. The effort brought me to tears on many mornings, but I was always encouraged to keep trying. Betsy explained,

"Each day your coordination is improving, Carole. You just have to keep trying."

"I can't even dress myself," I cried as I toppled sideways onto the bed.

"Don't give up now. You are making progress," Betsy urged as she pulled me back to a sitting position and handed me the stick for another try.

Betsy was right, I knew, but she may not have realized how utterly frustrating it was to be unable to dress myself. A toddler learning new tasks has no idea of the possibilities or the limitations. While my skill level was that of a toddler, I knew exactly what the right movements were. I just couldn't execute any of them.

As days turned into weeks of practice, Betsy watched me struggle, offering helpful hints, until she knew I was too exasperated to continue. Then she'd help with just the right placement of a piece of clothing or a tug where the elastic needed an extra stretch to fit over my hips. Each day I seemed to do a little better, but it would be months before I could dress myself.

At every meal Betsy strapped a unique feeding utensil to my wrist then encouraged me to spear my food with the fork-like tines or scoop with the spoon-like part of this ingenious device. The easiest food to manage was mashed potatoes because it clung to the "spork" while Jell-O slithered right away from me. Once I had something on this feeding implement, I had to get it from the plate to my mouth. I could visualize how the spork should move, but my arm and hand muscles wouldn't always comply. Just as in dressing, this was going to take a lot of practice.

Wheelchair clinics were a necessary but depressing experience. All patients going home using a wheelchair had to be fitted for a chair and instructed on its use. Many people would use a wheelchair for life and were struggling to cope with the concept and skill development necessary to give them as much independence as possible.

As I had believed from my first days in the ICU, I still felt I would eventually walk again. Dr. L had talked with me several times about a mechanized wheelchair I could operate with a lever using my chin. He first mentioned this when I was unable to move my hands, had not yet stood on my own, and couldn't conceive of how I was going to learn to walk again. Even then I rebelled against this notion. Now that I had movement in my hands and was walking long distances, I saw no reason for a motorized chair. I thought when I went home I would be very close to walking on my own and that even a manual wheelchair wouldn't be necessary for long.

I may not be strong enough to maneuver a chair over the carpet at home, I thought, but for the short time I would need a wheelchair, someone would always be around to push me where I needed to go. And Petra was so enthusiastic about the progress I was making, I felt sure I would be walking on my own very soon. But Dr. L kept encouraging me to consider the mechanized chair.

"Look, Carole," he stressed, "You want to be as independent as possible when you go home."

"But we live in the woods. I won't go out in my wheelchair unless someone else is with me."

"When no one else is home, you'll want to be able to get around on your own. A motorized chair will let you do that."

Nothing I said seemed to penetrate his desire for me to have the best mechanized wheelchair. I appreciated Dr. L's caring, but after a while I began to wonder if the real diagnosis was grimmer than I was being told. Perhaps they already knew I wasn't ever going to walk again. After all, they continued to give me electromylegrams* to see if the nerves were repairing along their entire

---

* Medical Appendix. Electromyography.

length or if, in the progression of GBS, some of the nerves had been severed, destroying my ability to recover full movement. Why else would Dr. L insist on a motorized wheelchair?

He showed me pictures of various kinds of wheelchairs. He showed me wheelchairs in the physical therapy room and told me that in several weeks we would have to decide on the kind of chair I would buy so I could practice in the wheelchair clinics.

I kept trying to move Dr. L in my direction hoping for a lightweight model I would be able to roll once my arm strength was built up and my hands could grasp the wheel rims. He kept telling me I would need the chin lever because my hands weren't functioning.

One day in the physical therapy room I found out Dr. L had decided to proceed as he thought best. Glen, Katie, and Eric were all there helping me through the rehab regimen. I practiced lifting my legs while lying on my back on the therapy table. Over and over I repeated this exercise, readying myself for some walking. Petra wound Ace wrap around my shoes, then up behind my calves to keep my toes from dropping as I walked across the tiled floor.

I positioned the walker, being sure the wheel stops were locked in place. Then I grabbed Glen and Katie who were on each side of me and stood up. Once up, I grasped the walker to maintain my balance. While I took a moment to gather my strength and the will to walk, Eric loosened the wheel stops and said,

"Get going, Mom."

"Give me a moment. I'm almost ready," I said as I struggled for balance before taking off.

After a few hesitant steps, I walked slowly out into the room, balancing on the chest-high walker. My feet felt sluggish as they clomped along one after the other, but I made it across the room where I sat down on a mat table to rest, conversing with my children who made this work almost fun.

As we wound up the session, Dr. L came in and whispered to Eric. The two of them signaled to Glen as they left the room. Katie and I sat and chatted on the bright blue mat table not all that anxious to return to the hospital room, but knowing lunch would soon be waiting there. Most of the other patients had already left, and the aides were putting things back in order, ready for the afternoon session.

There was a commotion at the door and Eric came rolling into the room in a motorized wheelchair guiding it with his chin on a metal flange. His body was rigid. His arms rested on each side rail of the wheelchair, motionless. He looked as though he were a quadriplegic just learning to operate a new vehicle. My heart leapt into my throat. I felt sick to my stomach. I began to cry.

For all I had been through myself, nothing bothered me as much as seeing one of my children in a motorized wheelchair as though he were to be there for the rest of his life. What also struck me was the appearance of this kind of wheelchair. Essentially, I was being told I would be confined to a wheelchair for the rest of my life. I was devastated.

"No, no, no!" I cried as Katie tried to calm me down.

Dr. L, Betsy, Eric, and Glen looked stunned. They had planned this big surprise to show me the kind of wheelchair I was going to get and I was acting like a fearful child. I shouted,

"I don't want or need that kind of chair." In an irrational burst of explanation, I said,

"I want a simple, lightweight chair I can use until I can walk on my own."

Betsy asked tentatively, "Would you just like to try it out?"

"No. I don't want that kind of chair."

"Mom, you don't have to have this kind of chair if you don't want it," Glen volunteered.

"It's okay, Mom. They can get you a lightweight chair," Katie said, comforting me with her arm around my shoulders.

"Get Eric out of that chair right now," I sobbed, tears streaming down my face.

Whatever had motivated the drive to get me a motorized wheelchair was cancelled. It was never mentioned again. The next time we talked about a wheelchair, Betsy guided me through the catalogue and assured me I could pick a lightweight model that would be easy for me to handle.

In a few days, a manufacturer's representative measured me for the wheelchair and ordered it that day. When it came in, I attended wheelchair clinics and practiced rolling the chair on my own. By the time it got there, I could rest my hands on the wheels and push hard enough to propel the chair on a hard-surface floor. It rolled easily. I learned to propel the chair forward and backward, make tight turns, stopping when I wanted to.

Stu and I took the chair outside and practiced in parking lots and sidewalks around campus. This was going to work just fine for me. And in the meantime,

I was working every day to increase my time and distance walking around Dodd Hall. Someday I planned to donate this wheelchair back to Dodd Hall.

By this time each physical therapy session was devoted mostly to walking. I was going longer distances as my stamina increased. Eric was there almost every day helping Petra and me in whatever ways he could. She continued her exuberant encouragement, never failing to come up with incentives for progress and explanations of why one approach might work better than another.

One day as we were walking across the room, Petra explained how the muscles in the buttocks work to propel the leg forward. To show Eric where the motion came from and how to stimulate my legs to move, she pinched the area on his buttocks to give him the specific idea. Startled, Eric jumped forward with a surprised "Ohhhhhh!" and agreed that pinch would get anyone moving.

Although Petra had intended it as a clinical demonstration, she turned beet red as she tried to apologize and continue her explanation at the same time. As we all laughed merrily, I recognized a growing connection between the two of them.

No longer able to take me in the pool because of the toe surgery, Petra introduced me to the parallel bars where I could continue to develop my motor skills. She positioned me with one hand grasping each bar allowing me to walk along between the bars turning at each end and traversing the length again. Because I could manage this on my own, it gave me a different feel from when I was leaning on the walker.

After I was accustomed to working on the parallel bars, Petra and I worked side by side one day on the outside of the bars. I held on with both hands as we practiced squats. I could only bend slightly at the knees, but as with everything else, Petra had a way of pushing me to bend "just a little more."

This day, as I tried to "bend just a little more," my right knee buckled without warning. Losing my balance, I tipped to one side as my left hand slipped off the bar. My other knee buckled and I sank toward the floor still grabbing the bar with my right hand. As my legs went into a full and complete bend, pain shot through both knees. Petra quickly grabbed for me as I spun out of her grip, shouting to Leon for help. The tendons and ligaments in my knees hadn't stretched that far in five months.

I screamed in pain and fear as I dangled from the bar. Leon came running from the far side of the room and helped Petra lift me upright from a semi squat.

This fall taught me a few things. I now knew the fear of falling. I had learned I couldn't pull myself up even though I had ahold of the bar. And if I had fallen all the way to the floor, I realized I wouldn't have been able to get myself back to a standing position. I still had a long way to go.

Poor Petra. I knew she felt terrible about the fall I had taken. But there is no way she could have kept my knee from twisting. Pushing for the outer limits of my capabilities risked occasional failure. And we found it. Besides, I thought optimistically, maybe that extra-tough stretch loosened up some ligaments and would make movement in my knees easier.

About this time, we started working on getting up off the floor. Backing off the two-foot high mat table, I edged one knee to the floor, then slowly lowered the other knee. From that position, I crawled toward Petra who had explained the technique of using a chair to pull myself off the floor. I grabbed the chair seat with both hands, brought one foot forward, pulling with my arms and pushing with my legs to get into a standing position.

Petra also soon had me climbing stairs. For two months I had watched other patients tentatively approach the four steps going up to a platform. On their first attempts, each of them struggled to lift one leg from the ground to the first step. Hoisting their whole body up just one step looked like torture and now, finally, it was my turn.

Indeed, when I was the one approaching the steps for the first time, I felt the challenge mocking me. I put my right hand on the right rail, left hand on the left rail and took a deep breath. I closed my eyes and tried to think how my legs were supposed to work to move me both forward and up.

I lifted my right foot and put it back down on the ground. I hadn't lifted it high enough to clear the first step. Once more I took a breath, lifted my foot as high as I could, just barely enough to slide it onto the first step. My arms pulled on the railings as my right leg strained at the hip to pull the rest of my body up to its level. Suddenly there I was with both feet on the first stair step. It was possible. Slowly I climbed the remaining three stairs and stood triumphantly on the little platform at the top.

"Great job Carole. Now, turn around and come down," Petra encouraged me.

I tried to suppress the anxiety I felt as I perched at the top of the stairs. It seemed impossible that I would be able to bend at the hip, knee, and ankle enough to lower my body to the first step. Coming up had been easy compared to this.

"If I propel myself too far forward I'll fall down all four stairs." I was paralyzed with worry. Petra knew the descent would be more difficult than the ascent, but she encouraged me nonetheless.

"Think about getting just one foot down. You can do it," she verbally pushed me forward.

"I'm afraid to lean too far forward."

"Don't worry. I've got you," she said as she tightened her grip on the safety belt around my waist.

I had grown to trust whatever Petra asked me to do. I knew she was strong enough to hold me if I faltered. As I hesitated, she prodded my heel gently from behind, moving my right foot toward the brink. It slid over the edge and I dropped down one step with my other foot and half my body hanging back on the platform. Pain throbbed in my thighs and hips.

I grimaced as I moved my left foot off the platform and down a step. Swinging my foot down wasn't as hard as raising it, and finishing the movement lessened the pain. Three more steps and I was standing at the bottom of the stairs – another achievement notched in my mental GBS notebook.

Soon four stairs were not enough of a challenge and we went to a back-exit stairway where Petra had me climb ten stairs, then twenty. Soon I was feeling quite comfortable making my way up and down stairs, great practice for the stairs I would soon face at home.

Preparation for my homecoming was underway. Carpenters had built ramps and railings throughout the house reminding me of my severe limitations. I had come so far, but I still could not walk without a walker. I could climb stairs but only with Petra holding onto a gait belt or my pants, letting me know she was there if I needed her support. The only positive thing I could see in those ramps and railings besides their utility was they were very rough and obviously designed to be temporary.

Walking with a walker or between parallel bars had great limitations. It didn't feel like regular, carefree walking. To give me free-form practice, Petra strapped me into an elaborate harness suspended over a treadmill where I walked on my own, swinging my arms, with no one holding me from behind. She started the treadmill slowly, then increased the speed as I moved my legs faster.

About this time, Eric began questioning me about Petra.

"Do you think Petra is dating the tall, dark-haired physical therapy intern?"

"I don't think so. She's responsible for Mark's training."

"She spends a lot of time with him."

"Yes, I know. But that's because she's training him."

Eric shrugged and dropped the subject. I wondered why he was asking these kinds of questions. Eric was a confirmed bachelor.

At the same time, Petra was sharing some personal information about herself. She talked about her mom and dad who lived in Colorado Springs and told me some about her childhood, high school, and college years. I was getting to know Petra as a real person and not just my physical therapist.

For a while now, Betsy had attached me with straps to various machines, then had me pull or push, according to the purpose of each machine. Once I had gained some range of motion and muscle strength, I could grasp the handle bars on the machines, opening a world of more demanding therapy for my hands and arms.

Betsy also taught me practical things. In the computer room I practiced keyboarding, trying to redevelop my lost skills. She equipped me with braces to hold my hands rigid. I reverted from my former speedy keystroking to hunt and peck, using my index fingers to type out simple messages.

Betsy encouraged me to type a few lines to show Stu the progress I was making. The brief note on a pink sheet of paper showed both my progress and how far I still had to go. As it slid out of the printer, I read,

DEAR BSTU,B

THIS IS MY FIRST ATTEMPT AT TYPING A LETTER WITH MY HAND DEVICE. IT IS NOT AS DIFFICULT AS I EXPECTED. IT IS SLOW AND MY ARM IS STRAING TO KEEP FROM COLLAPSING ON THE KEYBOARD. NEW MUSCLES TO TRAIN. I WILL PRACTICE I WILL BE ABLE TO GO FASTER.

In my public relations job, I had spent hours at the computer hammering out meeting reports, strategic marketing plans, and other voluminous documents. It seemed so easy then, but now it was a challenge just to get two simple sentences on paper.

Stu had posted a sign in my room when I first went to the ICU. It said, "ONE DAY AT A TIME." We were going to advance one day at a time so as not to be overwhelmed by the magnitude of the challenge. It was still that way all these months later.

By now I had given up any thought of returning to work. I couldn't imagine living a normal life where I could move about my house, cook a meal, or entertain friends. These kinds of thoughts depressed me even though I knew I was making rapid progress. I still relied on the psychologist's visits every afternoon to pull me out of my self-pity, help me to realize how fortunate I was, and to be more practical about my expectations.

Now that I was close to going home, I gave a lot of thought to how my family and Petra had helped me get this far. For all these months, Stu's cheerfulness never failed in my presence and his devotion and advocacy never diminished.

Eric and Bonnie never missed a day of uplifting visits. While for them it must have seemed boring, their never-ending search for ways to entertain and console buoyed me through the roughest times.

Once Glen overcame his abhorrence of the hospital environment, he visited more often. Usually he was quiet but every now and then he'd crack a joke or tell a good story and punctuate the moment with a dimpled smile and a twinkle in his eye.

Katie sacrificed most of her last semester in college to be home on weekends to help Stu and cheer me. And once she got back from her trip to Europe, she came often to Dodd Hall helping me learn how to function again.

By now I felt a firm bond with Petra. She was always cheerful and very aggressive with my therapy, pushing me farther each day until I was on my feet and could finally believe I would be going home.

Without the devotion of these six people, the arduous journey from February until now would have been unbearable. Only with their help was I able to recover enough to head for home.

On July 11 with the promise I would return for two weeks of "day hospital," Stu packed up my few belongings. We did a well-executed board transfer from bed to wheelchair, emphasizing this critical skill I had learned. As I waved, "Goodbye," Petra tucked a piece of paper among my things. In typical Petra fashion, it said:

Yippee! The chorus of everyday working with you.
Every now and then there is that extra connection
that keeps me thinking, wakes me up in the middle

of the night with "Oh! Let's try that!" Looking back at
where we started, it is amazing and exciting. I more
than look forward to where we will go! Congratulations
Carole, you are going home! Your courage and
determination are admirable and contagious. I am so
thrilled to be able to work with you.

Petra sent me home with a gift beyond measure: the hope that I might eventually be one of the 80 percent who recovers 100 percent.

Chapter Fifteen

Half Way Home

Waking up at home on Saturday morning brought a rush of questions about how I was going to function here without all the help I had at the hospital. First, Stu sat me up, then after we worked a pretty slick transfer into the wheelchair, I rolled into the bathroom. Stu offered to help with my morning ritual, but I insisted I wanted to do it myself, even if it was a struggle.

"Go make some coffee. I'll be out soon."

"See you in the kitchen when you're ready," Stu said, with a soft pat on my shoulder.

Grabbing the sink, I pulled myself to a standing position, found the toothbrush and started brushing. Next, I managed a few quick strokes of a brush through my hair. Because my elbows still wouldn't straighten, my reach was too limited to do a good job. Some lipstick. This wasn't an elaborate ritual yet, but I was in my own bathroom taking care of a few of my basic needs.

Using the dressing stick, I sat in the closet piling pieces of clothing on my lap. Was this the morning I could get a shirt on by myself? Nope. No matter what contortions I tried, my shoulders and elbows still refused to conform to the shape of a shirt. I slowly turned the wheelchair and rolled into the bedroom where I tried to loop pants over my feet and with only minor trouble stood, held on to the night stand, and pulled them up.

Leaving the shirt in my lap, I reached toward my feet to put on socks. My right hand brushed the top of my ankles draping a sock across my foot, but the muscles and tendons in my back and arms were so tight, I couldn't bend enough to put my toes in the sock. So, before he left for work, Stu finished dressing me. A frustrating disappointment.

My sleek wheelchair almost glided on its own that afternoon as I rolled up to the refrigerator, planning to make a sandwich. I pulled out the bread and swiveled to put it on the counter. Mayonnaise, lunchmeat, and lettuce followed. But my hands were too far below the counter to make the sandwich.

Slowly I pulled myself to a standing position. With a long stretch to the right I reached the flatware drawer, mindful that leaning too far would land me on the terra cotta tile floor. After unscrewing the mayonnaise jar lid, I quickly made the sandwich, then repositioned the chair so I could sit down. Oh, I forgot the plate. Too exhausted to get across the kitchen to retrieve a plate, I pulled a square of paper towel from the roller, grabbed the sandwich, and rolled slowly down the ramp into the great room.

Rolling on plush carpet was much harder than on kitchen tile, but pushing hard, I worked my way to the far side of the room. After I put the sandwich and paper towel on the couch, I pushed myself up to a standing position, executed a half-turn and let myself drop into the comfort of the cushions, just missing the sandwich when I landed. Making lunch felt like a huge accomplishment.

Following a short nap, I sat in front of the computer screen, resting my hands on the keyboard, willing myself to practice. I couldn't get out a one-page document without a multitude of errors, but practiced one page after another wishing Betsy were here to encourage me. "Not as good at this as sandwich making," I thought.

At night after dinner, Stu and I emptied a kitchen drawer, built dividers, and divvied out the assortment of pills the attending physician had prescribed when I was released from the hospital. We counted out anxiety reducers, mood elevators, stool softeners, blood thinners, and painkillers. So many pills to help me cope with all the complications of GBS. I wondered if I'd ever be free of them.

On Sunday I was determined to get out of bed by myself. I had practiced this every day at Dodd Hall, but now here at home, I just rested on my right side, unmoving as I couldn't think what I had to do to raise my body up.

Let's see, what did Petra tell me to do? Oh yes,

> "Scoot close to the edge of the bed then place both hands on the mattress near your upper chest. Okay, now push yourself upright while swinging your legs out of bed."

I tried once. Not enough push. Okay it takes a strong steady push at the same time coordinating the leg swing. After a few tries, I got to a sitting position. But now I couldn't do anything until Stu helped me with a board transfer to the wheelchair. He was out in the kitchen making coffee, so I waited.

And waited. I couldn't do much without someone else's help. Soon, with a cup of coffee in each hand, Stu was there to help with the transfer.

On Sunday we decided to relax and celebrate surviving five months of hospitalization. Together Stu and I practiced our new routines and figured out how we were going to adjust to our changed circumstances. We reminded ourselves that, really, it was only a long weekend at home as I would be returning to Dodd Hall on Monday for two weeks of Day Hospital.

✳ ✳ ✳

Katie was a big help this first weekend at home. With an efficient air and a can-do attitude, she helped me undress in the evenings and patiently helped me transfer to the elevated toilet as if she had done these things all her life. She gently wrangled with my clothes, getting them down and up just as handily as the therapists. Although it was hard for me to accept her help in such a personal function, it didn't seem to faze her and as the days went by she made me more comfortable with my limitations.

Katie also encouraged me to practice walking, usually initiated with a cheery command,

"Okay, Mom, let's get going. Stand up."

I had to think about it every time because no movement was automatic.

"First, lean forward," I rehearsed the procedure aloud,

"Then push with my hands and thighs and grab the walker."

Katie waited patiently, not saying a word. It took several tries but eventually I was standing.

"Now walk," Katie coached, I'm right here behind you with the chair if you think you need to sit down."

We walked from foyer to kitchen and back many times, building muscles and my confidence at the same time.

Monday morning I was back at Dodd Hall, almost as though I'd never left. Eric wheeled me to my old room where my bed was waiting for me, but Evelyn suggested I sit in the wheelchair and wait for Petra who arrived a few minutes later and took me to the therapy room.

Before beginning our routine, Petra explained that she and Betsy would now elevate our occupational and physical therapy goals and use morning and afternoon sessions to make as much progress as possible. There would be a short rest period at lunchtime and following the afternoon therapy session, I would be given an intravenous dose of IVIg.

The insurance company had granted me the extra two weeks and we were all determined to make the most of it.

After this brief explanation, Petra took me to the center of the therapy room to practice walking with a normal-sized walker. I pushed myself out of the wheelchair, then Petra guided me around the cavernous room, in and out of equipment, past other patients, most of whom were different from the ones I first met when I came to Dodd Hall.

By now I was climbing to the top of the back stairwell and down again. The range of motion in my ankles was increasing and I felt less pain than I had just the week before. The need to lean forward to move myself downward was still intimidating, but Petra, holding tenaciously to the safety belt, encouraged me with the ubiquitous "lean forward a little more."

After stairclimbing and long walks, we sat together on a mat table, discussing how to improve flexibility and strengthen my feet and ankles to overcome the foot-drop. Petra, in her usual practical way, suggested,

"Try to spell the alphabet with your feet."

"Really? With my feet?"

"It's easy. Just watch me."

After Petra traced the entire alphabet in the air with her right foot, I gave it a try. I did my best to form an A with my toes. Unlike Petra's effort, my letter wasn't recognizable, but Petra said,

"It doesn't have to look exactly like the letter, Carole, just keep moving your right foot in the form of each letter,"

I continued the drill until I couldn't hold my right leg up any more.

"Okay, Carole, let's try the left foot."

"I can't hold my leg up that long," I protested.

"Yes, you can. We'll take a break when you finish with the left leg."

Petra wasn't going to stop for fatigue or whining. As usual, she just switched to another body part to let the other recuperate.

While practicing this ankle-strengthening drill at home every night I thought of the day I would walk back into my office, so glad I had worn those Frankenstein boots for months to keep the foot drop from being worse.

I also pondered why no one during my five months of hospitalization had worked on my feet like they had on my hands. Because Gina spent two months on my hands at ATH and Betsy another two months at Dodd Hall, my hands worked well. So little had been done with my feet, though, that adhesions had formed between the many bones in each foot, making them feel like blocks of concrete clomping across the floor. What, I wondered, would have to be done to get them back to normal?

Lunch and a rest in bed prepared me for an afternoon session with Betsy. We did the usual work on my hands and shoulders then moved to a mock-up kitchen where I practiced meal preparation and a washer/dryer setup where I learned that this boring household task was within my power to accomplish on my own.

When occupational therapy finished for the day, I relaxed into the comfort of my bed, while Evelyn, using the port in my right arm, inserted the tube connected to a dose of IVIg. With a big sigh, I closed my eyes and enjoyed the good pain of exercise and felt the exhaustion of hard physical work wash over me.

The day-hospital routine was much the same Monday through Friday. In the second week, though, there was one unusual difference: Betsy asked if I wanted to practice driving. I was astonished. My hands were functional enough to grasp a steering wheel and I could sit up in the front seat of a car. But didn't people realize I couldn't feel my feet or know where they were in space unless I was looking at them?

The next afternoon a grandfatherly looking man with a fringe of curly white hair over his ears came into my room with Betsy.

"Hi, Carole. This is Charlie. He's going to give you your first driving lesson.

"Are you ready for this?" he asked. I said I was, but didn't feel at all confident.

With my agreement, Charlie pushed the wheelchair quickly down the long hall toward the elevator. As we exited the building, he leaned around from the back of the wheelchair, gave me a broad smile and cheerfully said,

"The car is over this way. Are you ready to drive?"

"I'm going to try," I said.

By now I could get out of the wheelchair and into a car on my own so I managed that first step easily. Charlie, adjusting his rumpled brown suit, got in the passenger side while he gave me a few instructions about this kind of car.

"Go ahead and drive to the far end of the parking lot."

Thinking it would be important for me to drive as soon as possible, I didn't mention that not only could I not feel my feet, but also, I could not guide them without looking at them. So, as I drove I glanced surreptitiously down toward the pedals to be sure my foot was in the right place.

When we got to the far end of the parking lot, I looked down again as I moved my foot to the left searching for the brake. Finding the pedals was one challenge, but I also had no sense of how much pressure I was exerting with my foot. I could push too hard on the gas and overshoot the end of the pavement or jam on the brakes instead of coming to a gradual halt. Why would anyone think I should be taking a driving lesson at this point?

We practiced several times that week, then Charlie announced I was ready to drive on my own. He asked if I wanted a permanent or temporary parking placard. I took the temporary one consistent with my expectation that I was going to be totally well at some point, but I realized it would be a long time before I felt safe driving a car.

Ten additional days of therapy showed in the progress I made. I was gaining more confidence in my ability to try things on my own and each day it seemed I could walk a little farther, type a little faster, and stay out of bed a little longer.

After therapy on the last Friday, I was in my room alone packing up a few things when I turned to sit down in the wheelchair, lost my balance, and toppled into the shower stall. My head crashed into the tile wall as I crumpled into a heap on the floor. Not hurt, but a little dazed, I looked around wondering how I was going to get to a standing position without a chair like I used in therapy.

A cord hung from the shower wall just like many I had seen in doctors' offices: just pull the cord if you need help. I gave the cord a tug. Within minutes six people were gathered around asking how I was and what made me fall and if I could get up on my own. Before I could consider that, Dr. L and several nurses pulled me to a standing position and suggested I might want to sit in the wheelchair.

"We've been waiting for weeks for you to fall," said Dr. L.

"Oh really," I said, thinking this was an odd expectation.

"It's important for you to know you can fall and not get hurt."

Well, this had been good practice because it hadn't hurt at all.

With this last lesson from almost two and a half months at Dodd Hall, I wheeled the chair back into my room to wait for Stu. We were about to begin a new phase of recovery, one we would navigate without the help of the caring therapists, nurses, and doctors at Dodd Hall. Then I caught a glimmer of hope that all contact with my therapy team would not be lost when Petra quietly asked,

"Would it be alright if I asked Eric for a cup of coffee now that you are no longer my patient?"

Chapter Sixteen

Finding My Former Self

B eing home for good was a challenge, but a good one. My days were filled with the promised outpatient therapy back at OSU, a daily visit from an infusion therapist to continue IVIg treatments, practice stretching and walking on my own, and struggling with all the day-to-day tasks that were still so hard to do.

On my first visit to Ohio State University's outpatient therapy program, I was struck by its size and the amount and kinds of equipment arrayed against the walls. Each activity center was freshly painted in bright, cheerful colors. It made Dodd Hall look like an old, worn out high school gymnasium.

Two young therapists greeted me at the reception desk and took me right to work on a modified treadmill with a harness to hold my body upright while I improved my walking speed. Sally, a tall lithe blond, clipped the harness buckles while Ann explained how this exercise would work.

"Hold on to the handrails, here," Ann instructed.

"I'll start the machine slowly so you can get your stride. The harness will hold you up if you lose your footing." Sally joined in,

"This will help you walk faster and improve your gait."

I relaxed, walking as naturally as possible, and when I tripped, I just sank a little until the harness caught me. A quick scramble and I was back on my feet without having to stop the machine.

Eric drove me to the medical center three days a week for three hours of therapy. While Ann and Sally did some work on my hands and arms, they concentrated most of their efforts on walking and balance.

One particularly challenging device required me to stand on a board about eighteen inches wide and four feet long. It teetered from side to side like a miniature seesaw and, also moved back and forth. It was challenging to maintain my balance while Ann manipulated the board through various positions. What a great way to build my leg and ankle muscles while gaining some control of my own balance. It was like being inside a video game or snowboarding down a mountain slope.

Oh, what Petra could do with equipment like this!

Just as the new outpatient routine began to settle for all of us, we learned that a dear friend had died in an automobile accident. Ruth was a beloved friend of many in Columbus, a legacy from years of professional and volunteer activities.

Determined to attend the funeral, Stu helped me dress up for the first time in seven months. He rolled me out to the car and with little help, I got into the passenger seat. Stu hefted the wheelchair into the trunk and, as we drove across town to the church, Stu wondered,

> "How do you suppose John is doing?" Ruth's husband was also well known and loved by so many in Columbus.
>
> "Surely, he's devastated," I said.

The parking lot was nearly full. People milled around outside the church, talking in hushed tones beneath overarching trees as we found our way inside.

Stu parked me in the wheelchair section, locked the brakes, and found his way to a regular pew. I looked up at the high, arched wooden ceiling where my eyes stayed during most of the service as I fought back tears, thinking of Ruth.

As the service came to an end, Stu released the brake on the wheelchair while commenting on the beauty of the service. Once outside, as we rolled slowly toward the car, I saw people I knew from the Columbus business community, Children's Hospital, and my years of volunteer work. Not one spoke or even acknowledged they knew us.

I had heard about this phenomenon: healthy, able people don't "see" people in wheelchairs. This seemed impossible to me. How could people with whom I had served on boards and committees, attended symphony performances, and run 5Ks not "see" me? There was a lot about recovering from physical disability that I did not yet fully grasp.

✳ ✳ ✳

Not every day was filled with the strain of recovery. There were lighter moments, like when I decided Carole needed a relaxing bubble bath. Not since ATH had she soaked in a tub. The utilitarian "carwash" showers at Dodd were followed at home with the walk-in shower. It was about being clean, not relaxing.

My clandestine plan required shopping for a bubble solution with a nice aroma. One that would produce quality bubbles. I did not understand what a quality bubble looked like but I wanted nothing but the best for Carole.

I carefully prepared the bath. The directions were simple: "While running warm water into the tub, add 1 cp. full of solution. Fill the tub to desired level. Relax and enjoy." I made one minor adjustment. I reasoned that a deluxe bubble bath would require a little more bubble solution then recommended.

I turned on the Jacuzzi jets' timer and went to get Carole. Wrapped in her favorite bathrobe, she was sitting with comfortable anxiety in her wheelchair. We rolled into the bathroom where we worked together to get her into the tub. There seemed to be a lot of bubbles already even though the water wasn't very high yet. "Yep, this is going to be perfect," I thought.

"Relax and enjoy yourself," I encouraged. "I'll be back in twenty minutes or so."

Carole's smile let me know she was enjoying the moment almost as much as I was.

As promised, I walked into the bathroom twenty minutes later. Carole had managed to turn off the water, but there was no way for her to control the bubbles. They filled most of the room, floor to ceiling, wall to wall. I couldn't even see Carole's head, but I could hear her laughing.

"How much bubble bath did you put in here?" she sputtered.

"A cupful like the directions said," I offered. "or maybe just a little more than that."

"A CAPFUL, not a cupful!" she laughed.

I brushed enough of the bubbles aside to find Carole. She smiled at me in a way I had not seen in ten months. It was a look that made the roomful of suds disappear. A look that wrapped all the emotions together: love, appreciation, understanding, together with "Where did I ever find you?" It was the look I had seen as a teenager, when we got married, and a million time during our lives together. But, for the past ten months it had been absent. At that moment, a realization rushed through me,

"She's back!"

We both laughed as I got her out of the tub and into the shower to rinse off. Then she watched from the wheelchair as I used sheets to drag the roomful of suds outside to disburse them in the neighborhood. Physically, Carole still had many challenges, but the true Carole I had known all of my life was back.

❋ ❋ ❋

A week later I sat in a lounge chair on the deck looking out over the ravine. The summer's heat warmed my face as I waited for Petra and her friend to arrive for a first at-home physical therapy session.

Stu had asked Petra if she would come to our house to continue the kind of aggressive therapy that had brought me so far already. Petra agreed and suggested we also hire her long-time friend, Meg, a phenomenal occupational therapist and Lutheran pastor, who would work on my hands, elbows, and back while Petra focused on my hips, legs, and feet.

Petra and Meg, laughing and joking, came out to the deck with Stu. Petra introduced Meg, then guided me into the house with a buoyant, "Let's get to work!"

Exercises to strengthen and stretch my leg muscles were imperative as my walking was still hesitant and awkward. And, there would be no quickening of pace unless I strengthened my ankles and eliminated the foot-drop. So, we had to double the work on my feet. Petra got right to work with some familiar exercises and other new, more challenging ones.

Meg alternated sessions with Petra. Just as Petra and I finished a stair climb, Meg was ready with bone crushing maneuvers on my back.

"Yow, your shoulder blades are frozen in place. Do you feel this stiffness here in your shoulder?" Meg said in her boisterous and enthusiastic voice, her long, silvery grey and black hair falling over one eye.

As she pushed my right shoulder blade, trying to slip it over the underlying ribs, she met impossible resistance. Pain shot through my back and I let Meg know,

"It feels like my shoulder blades are glued to my ribs."

"No kidding? We are going to have to work hard on them," she acknowledged as she pushed more forcefully.

"Can they ever be loosened up?" I mumbled, my face pressed into the white carpet.

"Of course, but it's going to take a lot of painful work."

Meg could feel the reality for herself in the rigid resistance in my elbows and back. But she also knew her capabilities and was going to use them to free up every frozen part of me. It would take months of forceful manipulation to get my shoulder blades free.

"Lie on your stomach while I work on the left side."

"Okay," I agreed as I rolled over.

Meg twisted and pushed, rolled and manipulated my left side. The pain told me she was breaking things loose as I held my breath to keep shouts from spilling out.

Elbows were next on Meg's list. Little progress had been made with these joints. To get function back, adhesions had to be worked loose, so once the pounding, pushing, and forcing my shoulder blades and ribs were done, Meg stretched and twisted my elbows gently but relentlessly.

The three of us laughed and joked our way through months of therapy afternoons as we became better friends, both women forcing me toward greater mobility. My body responded to all the challenges Meg and Petra could think to offer and, week by week, I felt myself getting stronger and more flexible.

While I continued this organized therapy, I also practiced routine things like laundry, house cleaning, and cooking but like the slow, slow progress at ATH, I couldn't see much improvement here at home either.

Life aside from therapy reflected many other changes. Katie talked more often about joining Keith in Dallas where he was working with his brother Trevor in a computer warehouse. He had rented a house and was anxiously waiting for Katie to join him.

As the months moved into autumn I knew Katie's time with us was short. She needed to get on with her life and I needed to learn how to get along without her. It's bittersweet, seeing a child grow up and launch out on her own. She had found a wonderful, caring, thoughtful man and wanted with all her heart to be with him, not stuck in Ohio with her life on hold.

Eric and Petra's coffee date had grown slowly and steadily into more than just a casual friendship, but I couldn't quite tell how it was going. Neither of them was sharing their thoughts, but they continued to see each other almost every weekend. Eric still worked nights at the Ohio News Network while he completed his MFA. He, like Katie, was ready to relinquish caregiving duties.

Glen was now managing a busy and popular family restaurant in Columbus' downtown mall. He was a natural manager with a firm but caring manner with chefs, cooks, and wait staff. We knew he was still seeing Meri and, when they had time off together, they came to visit.

Stu knew better than I did that not only did I need to work every day on physical rehabilitation but also find ways to get my mind readjusted to a typical life. He decided it was up to him, personally, to work on my mental wellbeing. Not long after I completed day hospital, Stu announced that the first step in his plan would be a trip to our cottage on Chautauqua Lake.

Three months before Gullain-Barré Syndrome felled me, we had bought a small, white ranch house on a knoll overlooking Tinkertown Bay. For months the house sat, as if abandoned, in a small neighborhood of twelve houses nestled by the lake. Our neighbors must have wondered where we had gone after buying the property.

As I sat thinking about Stu's proposal to take a weekend trip, I knew it would be easy to spend two nights there. I happily agreed to the adventure especially because Stu's brother Don, and his wife Molly planned to join us.

On the four-hour drive, Stu stopped frequently to let me stroll around a parking lot while he held on to the back of my pants. I pretended to be a normal person as I tried to get the blood out of my feet and up toward my heart, an effort to relieve the pain in my feet.

As we drove off the main highway, I saw the shoreline, a flock of geese on the lawn, and the little white house. My heart lifted. We walked hand in hand up to the front door where I climbed three steps and walked into a house I barely remembered. The white tile floor in the entryway flowed into a living room on one leg of an L, the kitchen on the other.

"Sit here in front of the fireplace while I bring the suitcases in from the car," Stu offered.

"Oh, won't it be fun to think about redecorating this place?"

"Start making your plans," Stu encouraged me.

He was so right. This was a great way to get my mind off therapy and exercise. Here I could see one of the things I was fighting for.

The weekend reinforced my limitations but also raised my hopes. Stu stored the wheelchair in an out-of-the-way place knowing it would be impossible to use without wheelchair ramps. I would have to push myself to move in and out of the house on my own.

The next day Stu insisted on going down the hill to the dock. With help from Don and Molly, he encouraged me to embrace this outing to the shoreline. We would be closer to the ducks and geese. We might see fish swimming near shore. While a little part of me thought this might be fun, the whole idea worried me. I knew when he got me close to the water, that wouldn't be the end of this adventure. But I fixed what I hoped was a relaxed look on my face and held my breath as Stu pushed the wheelchair forward.

It was pleasant rolling down the hill toward the four towering willow trees whose branches hung out over the water. But when Stu wanted to roll me out onto the dock, my heart froze.

"No," I protested "I can't swim. Don't take me out there."

"You won't fall in," Stu persisted. And Don reminded me,

"Carole, the water's only a few feet deep under the dock."

Once out on the dock, Stu wanted to get me into the boat, something not that easy even for a totally able person. But with his usual confidence, he insisted I could do this. As he lifted me out of the wheelchair, I clung tenaciously to him, burying my head in the crook between his neck and shoulder.

Don lifted my feet over the gunwale and I sat on the edge waiting for Stu to climb into the boat. I held on until my knuckles turned white when he finally lowered me into one of the passenger seats. Don and Molly settled into their seats as Stu started the engine and carefully backed off the boat lift.

As we shot over the water toward Chautauqua Institution, I leaned my head back, closed my eyes and felt the spray of water on my face. It was like that day when the nurses took me outside at American Transitional Hospital. A special connection with nature. The joy of being alive. Fun with family. Stu knew what he was doing to push me this way.

✳ ✳ ✳

Every day sitting on the green sectional looking out at the thick woods beyond our house, I thought about past walks in the ravine and wondered when I would be able to walk there again with Smokey and Max. I was making so much progress now, but this particular joy was still out of reach.

Wonderful experiences were available, though, even without descending into the woods. One day, I noticed movement about thirty yards away on an upper branch of an enormous beech tree. Grabbing the binoculars, I focused them on a large barred owl and its fluffy white baby. As I watched this live

National Geographic special with amazement, the adult pulled a rodent into bite-sized pieces and fed it to the baby owl who sat stoically, moving its head from side to side.

Every evening after dinner as we settled down to watch TV, Stu gathered lotion and towels for a massage of my painful, aching feet. Although the extreme pain I had experienced throughout my hospitalization had lessened, the pain persisted from mid-calf down. Obviously, blood pooled in my feet as the day went along and needed to be massaged upward toward my heart. This and ice packs were the best remedies we ever found for this lingering pain.

As September flipped into October, Stu asked me to consider attending the annual meeting of one of his favorite healthcare groups in Colorado Springs. I felt I could probably manage the trip although most of my moving around would still require the wheelchair.

The first surprise was the airline's preparation for handling passengers in wheelchairs. It was easy to arrange transportation of my own chair and an airport attendant was always available with one of theirs to wheel me to my destination while Stu handled the luggage.

Unlike our experience at the funeral, long-time friends at the conference welcomed us with questions about my progress and what our plans were for the future. We participated in all the group activities and thoroughly enjoyed ourselves.

Stu so wanted me to feel back to normal even if I wasn't quite yet. Walking around the hotel's beautiful grounds is something we had done many times in the past and Stu wanted me to try it now with my developing abilities.

"Let's leave the wheelchair in the room and just walk slowly over to the pond," he suggested.

"I can't do that, Stu. I don't have the strength."

All I could imagine was getting a hundred feet from the hotel and not being able to go another step further. I don't think he understood I still had significant limitations. Pushing me was so beneficial, but I had to reintroduce the realities of my recovery over and over again.

"I'm making progress, but I'm not ready for this walk yet."

We compromised. Stu brought the wheelchair along and I walked as far as I could without it. More than an hour passed as we moved through the pines and past the pond where we found a woodcarver at work on a gnome. After chatting for five minutes or so, I tugged at Stu's sleeve and requested we start back toward the hotel where I could rest before dinner.

Four days away removed me from the comfort of routine. It challenged me to come up with solutions to new problems and to figure out how to accomplish what I needed on my own. When Stu was at meetings, I got myself up and dressed. I walked around the hotel room on my own, without support from behind. I ate among friends at upscale restaurants without the aid of adapted flatware. This was one of the biggest challenges, proving in the end that I could eat normally and not spill dinner in my lap.

My sister, Barbara, must have had similar thoughts to Stu's. With her experience as a travel agent and desire to prod my slow improvement, she planned a girls' weekend at a resort in central Pennsylvania, a treat for Mom and her three daughters. The Colorado trip had pushed me to the limit, but I thought I would be able to manage another weekend away with Barbara driving and handling all the details.

While I looked more normal than I had in the hospital, looks can be deceiving. Not wanting to complain constantly about the pain in my legs, feet, and hands, I kept quiet, trying to force it into the background as we enjoyed the spa, dinner in the lodge and nearby restaurants, and just relaxing together and talking. I tried not to show my fear of walking in public without wheelchair backup. But the fear of falling nagged my every step. Each night as I drifted into sleep, I thought how hard it was to be "normal" yet silently thanked my caring family for pushing me so hard.

✳ ✳ ✳

The last few months of the year rolled by in a blur of therapy, increasing tasks accomplished on my own, and thoughts of returning to work. With all Meg's work loosening my elbows and back I was now able to pull a shirt over my head. I could put on my own underwear and slip my feet into comfortable shoes. I could not, however, reach my feet and put on a sock. While standing, I still could not lift one foot into a pant leg, followed by the other one. I had to hold on to something for support.

Sandy was working out the details for my return to work in late January. She negotiated with the long-term disability insurance company for me to return to work 80 percent time to see if I would be able to manage the workload. I wondered if I was ready.

There were still many limitations. I was unsteady on my feet. My keyboarding was slow. And I was taking naps every afternoon. Only getting back to work, I thought, would push me past these barriers.

Every December Sandy hosts a holiday party at a downtown club. Stu and I were invited to the upcoming one, a chance to see my colleagues and former clients, to enjoy social interaction, and to begin to slip back into my old world.

As we walked up to the looming stone building in the dark, Christmas lights twinkled on the wrought iron railings and over the front doorway. Stepping out of the cold winter air into the warm interior, we felt the warmth of friendship mingled with the smell of roast beef, chicken, and shrimp appetizers. People flowed through the first-floor rooms, balancing plates and drinks while conversation buzzed in competition with the sound of Christmas carols. It was energizing to talk with so many people and to think about returning to work in about a month.

Chapter Seventeen

Am I There Yet?

New Year's Eve was cold and crisp. Snow fell softly through the thick woods behind the house and swirled into drifts on the deck. We sat together, Stu and I, a fire roaring in the fireplace as we thought of the year to come and what was in store for us and for those who had helped me through my struggle with GBS.

Katie and Keith would be back from a trip to Portugal in a few days, then head for Dallas where they both planned to work in the computer warehouse. I wondered, but hadn't asked, how this fit with their college degrees. I hoped living together would move both of them toward marriage and permanent career choices. I hadn't mentioned that either.

Bonnie continued her work as a custom framer for Michael's where her artistic talents were put to good use, but her best gifts were more useful at her second job at the James Cancer Hospital providing art therapy for children whose parents had cancer.

Eric's next career moves were certainly on the horizon and, hopefully, he was factoring Petra into the equation. I wondered what they might be planning.

Glen and Meri had moved in together in the fall and he encouraged Meri to follow her dream of a college degree in human resource management which she was pursuing at a local university.

I looked forward to the coming year with some excitement but even more doubt and fear. Returning to work had been one of my major goals and now I was going to test my readiness. I could walk alone with a four-pronged cane. Eating was no longer a problem. My keyboarding skills continued to improve. I felt ready to meet my staff and learn how things had changed while I was in the hospital.

What I was less ready for was meeting new clients, taking charge of their public relations plans, and aggressively recruiting new business. All of this would require active engagement in the business community, getting around town by walking and driving, and entertaining new prospects.

All these thoughts swirled through my head like the snowflakes outside. I felt indecisive and panic stricken. The best I could do was show up for work and figure things out one day and one challenge at a time.

As the second hand swept past midnight, Stu and I hugged tightly, then he brushed a loving kiss gently across my lips before pulling me off the couch and directing me toward the bedroom. The New Year stretched out before us as we settled into bed and wondered what the next twelve months would hold.

✳ ✳ ✳

Two days later Katie and Keith returned from Portugal, bursting with exciting news. While Stu and I had enjoyed a roaring fire on New Year's Eve, Keith was proposing to Katie in Lisbon. She excitedly showed us the ring and chatted about our trip to Dallas at the end of the week when we would help them settle into their first home.

After two and a half days of flat, bleak, winter terrain, we drove into a Dallas suburb and pulled up to a modest ranch house. Frequent rest stops and understanding companions made the trip easier than I had expected.

The next two days were a hectic and stressful time for everyone as we helped clean up after an unanticipated flood and organized their possessions in the little grey ranch house. Katie remembers,

> "Dad wasn't ready to leave me there in Dallas and you were still recovering physically and emotionally. I just wanted silence to perfect my plan for setting up my first home with Keith and his dog, Christine."

She also remembers an argument between the two of us, the subject of which neither of us remembers, during which I announced I was leaving the house on my own. As I moved slowly down the sidewalk, Katie observed,

> "There goes mom, storming away at the pace of a tortoise."

Stu suggested she follow me, but Katie, knowing me well, wasn't having it.

> "I think it would be better to let her cool off."

When Katie did get in the car sometime later, she found me just three houses down the street, still steaming. She might not have realized that while I was furious at whatever the issue was, I was happy, at least, to be storming away on my own.

This episode reflected my emotional state six months after my discharge from the hospital. My emotions were always at the surface and hard to control. I was tense and still fighting constant pain. Everyday tasks, like walking and eating, demanded my full attention. When an unexpected task popped up, it felt overwhelming. At the time, I didn't correlate this lack of ability to cope in everyday life with the challenges of returning to work, but I should have.

* * *

The third week in January, eleven months after the onset of Guillain-Barré Syndrome, I returned to work. Eric drove his green pickup truck up to the loading zone in front of the familiar high-rise. As traffic whizzed by, he helped me out of the passenger seat, retrieved my cane from the flat bed, and gave me a squeeze as he said, "Good luck, mom. Go get 'em," while guiding me toward the revolving door.

I hadn't thought about wrestling with a revolving door. As Eric climbed back into the truck and drove away, I approached the door. People were rushing in and out as it whirled so fast I couldn't imagine how I would be able to move through it. I stood to one side trying to calculate how to step into the pie-shaped space without catching the cane in the door or tripping on one of my feet. I also wondered how I would push the door while working the cane. And how could I stop the door from pushing me from behind when I wanted to exit? They didn't have a practice revolving door at Dodd Hall.

Suddenly a lull in foot traffic gave me the chance to move into the slowly revolving door without anyone else pushing. I walked slowly, the cane tucked under my right arm, then exited with no trouble at all. I closed my eyes briefly before starting the walk across the marble floor to the bank of elevators. All of this felt so new to me. It wasn't just "going back to work."

People were gathering by the elevators, carrying briefcases and cups of steaming Starbucks. The aroma reminded me of work days long gone when I would have had one in my hand on the ride to the 20th floor. But today it would take every bit of concentration to get me up there without coffee or a briefcase. The cane and a purse were all I could manage.

Things looked just as they had last February as I walked slowly from the reception area down a long corridor of work cubicles to my office. Few people were in yet, but Sandy greeted me warmly and took the last few steps with me into the office.

"Can I get you a cup of coffee, Carole," she asked, "while you settle in?"

"Oh, that would be great," I said, glad I wouldn't have to figure out how to carry a cup of steaming hot coffee safely back to my desk.

"Do I remember correctly she asked," as she turned to go, "cream and one sugar?"

I responded with a nod and an appreciative smile. Sandy made me feel welcome and happy to be back. When she returned with an azure mug of steaming coffee, she said,

"There's a staff meeting at 9:00 am and everyone is anxious to see you." Placing the mug on the desk, she exited with,

"See you then."

A little trill of fear whirled around in my chest. How was I going to keep up with the chatter about new clients, prospects, and the week's workload? I felt overwhelmed and the work day hadn't even begun. "Take one thing at a time," I told myself, trying to calm my fears with the mantra we had used for most of the last year.

The office looked sterile. Everything that had made it mine was gone. The bookshelves were empty. The desk gleamed from its overnight polishing and two notebooks rested on the corner of the desk suggesting volumes of work inside. Placing the cane in a corner, I sat carefully in the swivel chair and got started.

The first day flew by in a kaleidoscope of colors, sounds, and emotions. People were welcoming and didn't dwell too much on what I had been through. They focused on helping me learn about current clients and advising me about the week's work. I tried to jot notes, but I couldn't write fast enough. I tried to read those notebooks when I was alone in my office, but my mind wouldn't seem to focus.

Someone saved me the worry about what I would eat for lunch by offering to bring in a sandwich from the deli down the street. I jumped at the offer, not wanting to venture out on my own just yet.

Early in the afternoon, I decided to visit Beth, the IT manager, at the far end of the office. I left the cane leaning against the wall. I didn't need it for this short walk. Foot drop still plagued me, so to keep from tripping on my toes, I lifted each foot a little higher than I used to.

And I wore clunky oxford style shoes with crepe soles as suggested by my neurologist. They were ugly and obvious, but they gave me stability. So, off to Beth's office I clomped, my eyes glued to the floor in front of me. I negotiated the long walk without much trouble.

As I entered her office, Beth came out of her chair with a big welcoming smile. Forgetting myself, I took one more step without lifting my foot far enough and dragged my right toe on the carpet throwing me forward toward the window. My reflexes were slow and while I saw the floor coming up toward me, I tried to take a few steps to catch myself. The whole episode proceeded in slow motion. Left step, right step. "Oh, no. You are going to hit your head on the window sill." I could also see Beth's horrified expression as she took two steps forward to try to catch me.

Somehow, I righted myself with a final grab at the window sill and did not go down. My heart pounded in my chest. I could feel the heat in my face. I couldn't talk. Beth graciously offered me a seat, saying,

"Let's sit together and talk."

"Thanks, Beth," I muttered as I tried to collect myself.

As we talked, my pounding heart returned to its normal rhythm. I apologized and admitted to Beth there were a few things about returning to work that were going to be difficult. Later, as I walked back to my office, holding on to the work cubicles as I went, I chided myself, "You should always use the cane."

* * *

Three months flew by as I tried to adapt to being in a work environment without all the skills I needed. This was so unlike my previous life when I went in early every day and often stayed late. Back then I could multi-task easily: talking on the phone, taking notes, and keyboarding a report.

Now exhaustion overcame me around 2:00 o'clock and I fought to keep a focus on work until Eric came for me at 4:00 pm. My schedule was dictated by my morning and afternoon rides. By pain and exhaustion. By working on just one thing at a time.

I went on a few client calls and even pitched a few prospects. One such effort always reminds me how difficult this time was.

Three of us went to the national headquarters of a fraternity coping with numerous negative campus incidents. They needed a comprehensive crisis management plan and we were there to pitch our expertise in hopes of securing the contract.

Their offices were in a large Victorian home where climbing the stairs to the front door seemed to take forever as I wrestled with my cane and tried to lift my feet high enough to top each step without tripping. My two colleagues were patient, but it must have seemed an eternity to them until I made it all the way up to the large porch.

Once inside we were greeted by the fraternity's committee members and asked to go up to the second-floor conference room. "Oh, no," I thought, "More stairs." The necessity of government requirements to accommodate the physically handicapped crossed my mind.

The stairwell was narrow, steep, and winding. With people in front and behind me, I held onto the wall taking the steps one at a time. When I stepped onto the landing, I took a deep breath, then walked slowly to the conference room where I slipped into an over-stuffed leather chair. I felt like everyone was looking at me. Were they wondering what was wrong with me?

But no one said anything and after brief introductions our staff began the presentation. Luckily, I was not the first to speak. As Amy explained our approach to crisis management, my mind wandered. My legs and back ached. I thought about how I was going to go down those stairs.

"Carole, why don't you explain our firm's qualifications."

My mind snapped back to the table. I could talk about the firm easily because I had done it many times before. The words flowed out automatically while I tried to give them emphasis and personality.

As we drove back to the office, we thought our chances of getting this client were good. And we were right. Despite my wretched performance, we won the contract.

That afternoon on the ride home I told Eric,

"I have no business being back at work."

"Don't worry so much, Mom. You can handle it."

"But I can't do even the simplest things." Wisely, he said, "Everyone knows you're still recovering. Just take it easy."

Nothing about venturing back to work was going to be easy. The long-term disability insurance company inquired in March about when I would be ready to work full time. They wanted my neurologist to confirm my continuing disability which I hoped he would do after my next appointment in April.

∗ ∗ ∗

Tired of my clunky oxford shoes, I put on light-weight black flats for my visit to Dr. M's office. Stu drove me to the medical complex and guided me to the fourth-floor office, optimistically leaving my cane behind in the car.

Dr. M greeted us warmly and escorted me into his office where he checked my reflexes just as he had done so many times over the last 14 months. He pronounced me "100 percent recovered" and then asked why I was wearing such flimsy shoes.

> "I'm tired of wearing the old boxy looking ones. I want to wear something fashionable."

> "You don't have enough strength in your ankles yet to wear that kind of shoe. It's dangerous. You still have foot drop."

So much for 100 percent recovery, I thought. If I still have foot drop, I am not 100 percent. But I didn't say that. Instead, I explained,

> "The disability insurance company is questioning my continuing need to work only 80 percent time. My boss needs your help to convince them."

> "I'll give them a call and assure them you cannot work full time yet."

Another indication I wasn't yet 100 percent, but I appreciated his reinforcing my continuing disability with the insurance company.

As we drove home I told Stu,

> "I think I should start weaning myself off all my medications, but I forgot to ask Dr. M."

> "Okay, when we get home we'll look at each prescription and make a plan."

Knowing I probably shouldn't quit cold turkey, we checked with my primary care physician, then set up a schedule and within two months I was drug free. In significant pain, but drug free.

Because I had been taking several pain medications for over a year, I minimized the reality of how much pain was still in my body. Once I swallowed the last pill, I realized I would have to adjust to constant pain and learn to live my life with it. It would take years for the pain to subside.

Chapter Eighteen

Beginning the New Me

While I struggled at work, I tried to maintain an exercise regimen at home. Except on weekends this was almost impossible because I was so tired when I got home in the late afternoon. But I did work on strengthening my ankles and walking without the cane every night.

Word had come from Dallas in late January that Katie and Keith planned to marry next October. As winter melted into spring, I thought more about wedding plans than work challenges and wished we lived closer to Dallas. Realistically, I knew Katie probably already had the outlines of a plan in mind, but I wanted to be involved as she worked to make her dreams come true.

Then Katie called to ask if I could fly to Dallas to help pick out her wedding dress. Barely thinking about taking days off work now that I had just returned, I jumped at the chance. Choosing a dress would be the beginning of her wedding plans and I couldn't wait to help. I figured a Friday through Monday trip would give me enough time without being gone from the office too long. When Sandy enthusiastically agreed, I booked my flights

Knowing Stu would take me to the airport and Katie and Keith would welcome me when I got off the plane in Dallas, I felt no qualms about making this trip on my own. Airline personnel were as helpful and courteous on these flights as they had been on our flight to Colorado Springs. As an attendant wheeled me into baggage claim, I saw Katie and Keith rushing toward me arms spread wide for welcoming hugs.

Shopping for the wedding dress was a special time. At several shops Katie tried on dress after dress. At the final stop, I rested in a chair while two women hovered over Katie, arranging the folds in each dress, pulling in the bodice to fit her tiny frame. It seemed like we looked at hundreds of dresses but none had seemed just right until Jasmine brought out a plain, flowing one with a scooped neckline and a subtle built-in train. It fit Katie almost perfectly and we both agreed, "This is the one!" As she swirled and turned on the elevated platform, I closed my eyes and sent up a silent prayer of gratitude that I could enjoy this moment with my only daughter.

As a sunny Texas dawn streamed in the window, I took slow steps to the suitcase resting on a chair in the corner and one by one slowly put on my clothes. The stretch to reach my feet was still a challenge. I leaned my chest down to my thighs trying to stretch enough to get the underpants looped over one foot. Three tries and I finally got it. Then I angled them toward the other foot. Same routine for the jeans. Thankfully, it was easier now to dress my upper half and I was soon ready to open the door and find my way to the bathroom.

After breakfast Keith and Katie drove me to the airport, and I winged my way back to Columbus. Relaxing my head against the tall seat, eyes closed, I thought about the rigors of this brief trip. Though I kept trying to appear and act normal, everything I did was still a struggle. I couldn't walk far enough yet to negotiate a large airport without a wheelchair. I couldn't stay on the go all day without having to sit down and rest. My legs and feet hurt all the time, making it hard to keep a smile on my face and a conversation going without showing the strain.

Recovery from Guillain-Barré Syndrome is a tedious drag. Dr. M's April declaration of 100 percent recovery didn't jibe with the condition of my body and the many things I was unable to do. Yes, I went to work every morning with hopes of a better performance, but my keyboarding was slow and my thought processes even slower. I rarely left the office for meetings or for lunch. I never returned to service on community boards that so interested me in the past. Not being able to drive pinned me to my office chair. And as the year moved on, I could still work only 80 percent time.

Petra and Meg's extra therapy sessions lasted until the end of March. Now Stu urged me to continue exercising on my own at a rehab facility about ten miles south of us, where I could walk a tenth of a mile track, holding on to a railing. Eric and Stu took turns accompanying me around the track, encouraging me to keep going when I said I wanted to go home.

One day as I walked through the door for a turn around the track, an old friend, coming out the same door, greeted me with,

> "Carole, I'm so sorry I didn't come to visit you when you were in the hospital."

> "Oh, that's okay, Cee, Stu let very few visitors in."

"I want you to know why I didn't come. My brother had a terrible case of Guillain-Barré Syndrome and I just couldn't face seeing you, knowing how his case turned out."

Cee's brother was a prominent chemist who was awarded a Nobel Prize shortly after his hospitalization. His case was so severe that many of his nerves were severed during the progression of the disease, leaving him paralyzed below the waist, the AMAN form of GBS that Dr. M had thought I might have. Cee recounted the excruciatingly difficult trip to Oslo for the ceremony, expressed gratitude that my outcome was so much better, then waved good bye as she headed toward the parking lot.

✳ ✳ ✳

At the end of July, Dr. M gave me a copy of a letter he had sent to the physician at the disability insurance company who was again questioning my continuing need to work only 80 percent time. As hard as I tried, it was not possible for me to work a full day. I felt guilty about this as I had been back at work for six months and thought perhaps I wasn't trying hard enough. Dr. M's letter erased any guilt I was feeling.

Dear Dr. B:

I received your letter...requiring further explanation for Carole W's disability....While she has made remarkable strides in your assessment, it should also be noted that she had a severe illness. She was completely paralyzed and on the ventilator as a result of Guillain-Barré Syndrome. I have managed patients who took more than three years to get back to any reasonable capacity for a full day's work....

The major problem Carole is now experiencing is that she has poor balance problems and that is not reflected in your assessment...It is not a surprise at all to me that a patient with this severe neuropathy would have poor large fiber function that would again take many months to return....it is also important to consider that patients with Guillain-Barré Syndrome take many months to recover any degree of stamina and ability to maintain even a sitting position for long hours throughout the day....I think it is remarkable that she is working thirty hours a week.

Sincerely yours, Dr. M

With this letter, Dr. M gave me a dose of reality. Someone probably should have counseled me not to attempt to return to work so soon.

* * *

The best parts of the year were those devoted to wedding planning. Just as she did in the hospital, Bonnie found hundreds of ways to sort through the details and negotiated key wedding decisions when Katie and I disagreed over one thing and then another. We couldn't have had such a unique and special wedding without Bonnie.

As the wedding day drew near, I was joyful. I felt comfortable, that holding Glen and Eric's arms I could walk the twenty-five yards down a slight hill to the gazebo next to the lake where Meg, the occupational therapist and Lutheran pastor, would perform the wedding ceremony.

Katie was beautiful in the sleek, filmy dress we had chosen in Dallas as she walked down the hill on Stu's arm to the strains of Pachelbel's Canon in D.

Keith in his tall hat and tails and the three bridesmaids in dark green with their escorts watched as Stu and Katie seemed to float down the hill. Despite all my worries about snow falling on this ceremony, the day was sunny and warm for the last day in October.

After the ceremony, Keith pulled our green canoe into the water, steadying it, as he helped Katie climb in. She tucked her wedding dress up under her and grabbed a paddle as Keith lodged his paddle in the rocky lake bottom to keep the canoe from rocking. They paddled south then swung west around the point, disappearing from view.

Yellow leaves still clung to the huge weeping willow trees surrounding the gazebo and I saw people wipe away tears as they watched Katie and Keith sitting tall through their dramatic exit.

I realized I was happier planning this wedding than working on any public relations plans. I felt more accomplished in the result. And I began to wonder more seriously if I should be working at all.

A debilitating case of Guillain-Barré Syndrome does more than attack the body. For me it shook my self-confidence. It diluted my concentration. It undermined my capacity to multi-task. And it left me with chronic pain that lurked at every meeting where I needed to pay close attention and under the desk when I was trying to compose a complicated report.

While life moves on, GBS clings to survivors and refuses to let go, and these lingering problems were affecting my ability to do the best possible work for my clients. This wasn't good for our team. Sandy needed a more capable vice president

I worked for months into my second year back, but finally decided it was time to face reality. Reluctantly, I ended my career, my community involvement, and my former professional self and turned toward an entirely different future.

❊ ❊ ❊

Weeks, months, then years flowed by.

I grew stronger and more confident. Occasionally, I dipped my toe back into the working world as when Sandy asked me to tackle a major writing project, a book-length report on how Ohio's police and fire departments designed a sophisticated statewide communication system for use during major traumatic events like tornados or terrorist attacks. Precipitated by the 9/11 attacks on the United States by Al Qaeda, the federal government gave each state money to improve their communications' capabilities. Each chose a different path and Ohio's proved to be one of the best.

The work spanned parts of two years and required me to visit with people in Columbus as well as leaders in police and fire departments around the state. I drove to those appointments on my own and as each was successfully completed, my confidence grew. The book was eventually published and distributed statewide.

Meanwhile Eric and Petra planned a six-month hike on the Appalachian Trail. Petra assembled hundreds of meals on our dining room table, boxed them up, and addressed each box to General Delivery in states along the entire route, their resupply system.

After work and on weekends they hoisted forty-pound packs on their backs and hiked up and down stairways in downtown parking garages building their stamina. One day at dinner they proposed that Stu and I climb with them more than halfway up Mt. Katahdin in Maine, the northernmost point on the AT and their chosen starting point.

> "Really, Petra, I don't think I can do that!" I pleaded, reminiscent of my reactions whenever Petra tried to push me beyond where I thought I could go.

"Oh, I'm sure you can. It won't be any problem and we'll have so much fun together."

Stu enthusiastically encouraged me to start planning for this adventure. I never climbed stairs in downtown parking garages, but I accelerated my walking, adding distance every day to get in shape for this adventure.

On a beautiful June day, we arrived at the base of Mount Katahdin. "What a monumental challenge," I thought as I looked up to the summit. The path started upward at a moderate angle, no rocks. But after an hour or so we were into boulders requiring Stu, Eric, or Petra to help pull me up and over the larger ones.

One foot in front of the other, I moved right along with the rest of them. By late afternoon we were at our destination, a campsite on the precipice Eric and Petra would scale the next day. We built a fire, enjoying the peaceful surroundings while organizing the lean-to, arranging sleeping bags on the wood floor, and preparing dinner.

I was so tired I never felt the wood floor of the lean-to beneath me. I fell right to sleep, not waking until 4:30 am when I heard swishing in the long grass uphill from our campsite.

I rolled over in my sleeping bag clutching it up under my chin as I leaned out to see a momma moose with her baby looking for breakfast. The hike to this point was worth every minute just to see them foraging for food in the subtle light of dawn. They were so close I could smell them. And hear their snuffling as they broke through the underbrush.

Hiking on Mt. Katahdin signaled the beginning of a new me.

Chapter Nineteen

Reflections

In a charming civil ceremony, the mayor of Westerville married Glen and Meri under a flowery bower in a small city park. Meri's parents, Stu, me, and two of Meri's friends, the only witnesses to a total surprise. Glen and Meri revealed this shocker when we showed up at their house to celebrate his birthday. Instead of the expected birthday luncheon, we all readjusted our expectations and joined the mayor for the ceremony at the park.

Just a week later, Eric and Petra married in the Hocking Hills forest in southeast Ohio, a silver lining that never would have been unveiled without the trial of GBS. Meg conducted the ceremony just as she had for Katie and Keith, an appropriate coincidence of the ribbons of Guillain-Barré Syndrome that brought us all together.

I have continued to make progress physically, emotionally, and mentally. With time, I have been able to reflect on my experience and consider how I might help other GBS patients, their families, and their caregivers.

When Petra became a professor at Ohio University, she asked me to talk with her first-year physical therapy students. The first time it was quite emotional for me to share my journey combating GBS, but the strong, positive response from students encouraged me to appear whenever Petra asked and to consider writing a book about my experiences in the hope of making a patient's struggles real to caregivers who might encounter people like me during their careers.

Stu took a job at Children's Hospital in Buffalo, New York where we enjoyed city life during the week and the restful Chautauqua Lake environment on weekends. Over time four more granddaughters joined Alex in semi-annual trips to the lake eventually learning to fish from the dock, drive the speedboat, and hike in the woods.

It took me five years to be able to pick a golf ball out of a cup on the green. It happened on a course at Hilton Head with a friend who had visited me with much apprehension at ATH, not knowing what to say to her friend who could no longer talk. We laughed about those days of fear and frustration as we walked to the next hole. And marveled about the simple things we take for granted, like bending far enough to retrieve a golf ball from the cup.

It took seven years before I could lower myself to a squat AND stand back up on my own. The pain lingered for years, but gradually concentrated in my feet where ice is still the best remedy after long hikes or a strenuous workout. Mostly I tried to ignore the pain so I could focus on all the challenging plans people hatched to keep me moving forward.

Seven years after Guillain-Barré struck, Eric and Petra; Katie and Keith; and my cousin and his wife, Steve and Susan, joined Stu and me on a 150-mile canoe trip. Chautauqua Lake spawns the headwaters of the Allegheny River and that is where we started paddling, with overnight camping on shore or on islands in the middle of the river. Our dream to paddle all the way to Pittsburgh was short-circuited by our fear of transiting the locks with large boats and barges, so we stopped at the charming town of Franklin where we rewarded ourselves with a night in a Victorian bed and breakfast.

Family and friends proposed all kinds of taxing stateside adventures and international travel. Stu and I have enjoyed two unforgettable trips to southern Africa where the culture, history, and animals seen on safaris captured our hearts.

Bonnie thought it would be inspiring to journey to Easter Island. So, we did, wondering often how Polynesians ever sailed in their reed boats to this most remote island on Earth. And why and how they built those towering statues?

Machu Picchu was even more inspiring and physically challenging. Stu persuaded me that I would be able to climb the steep, treacherous stairs and agricultural plains at 11,000 feet. And I did, with only modest difficulty.

Each of these trips stretched my physical abilities as well as my mind. They reminded me of the wonder of a world worth living to explore. And reinforced the importance of striving to regain normalcy no matter how long it takes. If I'd given up every time I'd wanted to, none of these things would have happened for me.

Some things never returned. I can no longer swim. I had to give up downhill skiing. I can't run any longer. But I can, and do, walk long distances. I lift weights and stretch on a regular schedule. I learned to snowshoe on the frozen lake and through the woods at our home in New York, one of Dr. M's suggestions. He thought snowshoeing would be much easier for me than cross country skiing.

There has been no end to the devastation of GBS on Carole's body that began on Valentine's Day weekend more than twenty years ago. In that cold Ohio February, we prepared ourselves for a battle that lasted weeks, then extended into years. We learned to endure the present, plodding day after day through excruciatingly minor improvements always yearning for a better future. We never consciously contemplated, "When will this be over?" In reality, it never will be over. There are many lingering effects.

Carole still deals with numbness and pain in her feet. She cannot feel where her feet are in space (a lack of proprioception) and, thus, suffers from instability especially if she is not looking down to know where her feet are going.

Occasionally, she laments her inability to multi-task the way she did before she was struck by GBS. However, her definition of multitasking is to handle about a dozen issues simultaneously, without missing a beat. Most people can't multitask like she used to, so I try to remind her that it's difficult to separate the slowdown of the normal aging process from the residual effects of GBS.

All in all, Carole has handled her changed life with the grace and determination that have always been part of her personality. The fact that she can only organize and process a few issues while she is preparing dinner with the assistance of five pre-teen granddaughters, a grandson and a golden retriever underfoot does not seem to register with her as a multitasking event. She still maintains high standards for herself.

We don't dwell on the grueling ordeal of GBS but rather the positives that came our way. At the very top of the list is our daughter-in-law, Petra. She not only changed Carole's life with a wholehearted approach to her care, she went on to change the lives of countless others by taking the energy that Carole and I witnessed directly into the classroom.

One of these classes wanted Carole to speak at their graduation dinner, a result of hearing her speak about her fight with GBS when they were first-year students. They especially wanted her to convey to their parents the importance of the profession they had chosen. To the students, Carole embodied what could be accomplished through thoughtful, dedicated, and quality physical and occupational therapy.

In her remarks Carole tried to express the importance of what they had learned in their course of study, but more importantly, how many people's lives they would change in the course of their careers.

Few things are more rewarding than the sincere, heartfelt comments from an entire class of young college students about to step into the real world as professional therapists. Their spokesperson addressed Carole directly from the podium,

> *"You have truly inspired each and every one of us. You reinforced why we wanted to become therapists. Deep down, we knew it, but we needed to hear it directly from a patient. You made it real. We will never forget the lesson you taught us."*

Anyone devastated by Guillain-Barré Syndrome must fight relentlessly to recover. For some the journey will be short. For others, perhaps as long a journey as mine. Looking back, I see several essentials to negotiating this arduous time.

When I close my eyes and think about those early weeks in the hospital, I am most grateful for Stu's encouragement, support, and love. He asked questions and pushed for answers when they were not forthcoming. He advocated for the best solutions for me. Not letting my eyes be taped shut. Not permitting the second toe surgery.

My own thoughts and actions as a patient were bound up in the actions of others. At the beginning, I would not admit that paralysis was taking over my body. I wanted to fight in every way possible. But when reality overcame my fortitude, I sank into a pit of black nothingness. I couldn't imagine how I would ever recover.

Reflecting now, I realize the importance of key caregivers. There were many, probably well-meaning, who still put obstacles in my way: Dr. R who didn't recognize the role of pain in causing anxiety; the resident who put me in diapers with a miscalculation on how to treat a minor urinary tract infection; the respiratory therapist who couldn't suction a mucous plug from my trach; and whichever person decided, or didn't decide, to treat my feet at ATH.

But there were many more without whom I would never have recovered: the attentive nursing staff on the ICU who pulled me through the weeks when I could have died; Ruthann, the caring, ultra-competent nurse at ATH who facilitated all my early progress like sitting on the edge of the bed and taking my first bath while giving me constant, loving care; Diana and Gina, the speech and occupational therapists who gave me the first glimmers of hope that I might get well, who got me talking and eating and who saved my hands; Phyllis, the world's best aide; respiratory therapist, Barbara, who wanted to help me get to Katie's graduation and who always provided top notch respiratory care; Tony and Leon at Dodd Hall whose every-day, joyful presence set the tone for rehab;

Betsy who worked diligently to make my hands and arms functional; and Petra, who saved my total being.

Underscoring family and professional caring was the constant flow of thoughts and good wishes from hundreds of people. There were those who came to visit like my boss, Sandy, and Professor L; Dr. T and Dean H, who didn't really have to; the gentleman at ATH who gave me as much consolation as he did his own mother; and the Ethiopian parking lot attendant who made the effort to find me.

I learned that recovery from Guillain-Barré Syndrome is a struggle unseen or unappreciated by most casual observers. People thought I looked well-recovered when I returned to work, but I wasn't. My balance was poor. I still had foot drop. I had trouble concentrating. The fatigue that caught me every afternoon was relentless. Even years later, unseen were skills that never returned, the continuing instability in my balance, and the pain in my feet.

Sometimes at night when I lie quietly thinking, I look at the little rag doll angel perched on the back of a loveseat in our bedroom. She reminds me that it is possible to make physical and mental strides long after professionals have advised that you have reached the limit of improvement. I imagine her winking as she remembers our long journey together from the ICU to now.

Medical Appendix

In Chapter Two

Deterioration of the Myelin Sheath

"The body's immune system responds to a perceived threat, like a bacterium, by producing antibodies to attack the invader. In Guillain-Barré Syndrome, the immune system perceives the body's own myelin sheath which covers the nerves, as a foreign body. Antibodies are produced that attack the myelin sheath, damaging it. This sheath acts as insulation on each nerve and enables signals from the brain to flow rapidly to the muscles. When the myelin sheath is degraded, the nerves cannot transmit signals to the muscles so the muscles cannot react. Nerves to the arms and legs are the longest in the body and, thus, weakness and tingling sensations usually appear first in the feet then later in the hands."[1]

What is Guillain-Barré Syndrome?

"Guillain-Barré (ghee' yan bah ray') Syndrome (GBS) is a rare autoimmune illness that progresses rapidly with symmetrical weakness in the extremities. This weakness is often preceded by tingling or pain in the legs."[2] "In many cases the symmetrical weakness, tingling, and pain spread to the arms and upper body. In the most severe cases, the entire body may be paralyzed. In these cases, the disorder may be life-threatening, requiring a ventilator and constant monitoring for abnormal heart beat, infections, blood clots, and high or low blood pressure."[3] "Two-thirds of patients report having a respiratory or gastro intestinal infection prior to the onset of GBS. A high proportion of patients with GBS experience pain. Approximately 25% develop respiratory

---

[1] Steinberg, Joel S. MD, PhD and Koski, Carol Lee, MD. "Guillain-Barré Syndrome, CIDP and Variants: An Overview for the Layperson." 2011, P. 5-7.

[2] Ibid, 2011, P. 3.

[3] "Guillain-Barré Syndrome Fact Sheet," NINDS. NIH Publication No. 11-2902, 2011, P. 1.

insufficiency requiring ventilation. About one-third of patients remain able to walk throughout the course of the disease, and are often described as mildly affected."[4]

In Chapter Three

Nerves that Control the Diaphragm

Nerves to the arms and hands exit the spinal cord from C5 to T1 (a reference to vertebrae in descending order from the skull down the spinal column; "C" is for cervical, "T" is for thoracic). When I reported tingling in my fingers, doctors knew the paralysis was still moving upward and would soon reach nerves to the diaphragm that exit the spinal column at C3 - C5. Without the use of my diaphragm, I would be unable to breath. Thus, the decision to perform the tracheostomy.[5]

A Brief History of Guillain-Barré Syndrome

"A French physician, Jean-Baptiste Landry, first identified GBS in ten patients of his in 1859. Each of these patients developed ascending paralysis from legs, arms, neck, and diaphragm over a few days or weeks. Landry found that in most patients their deep tendon reflexes (like that in the knee) were non-responsive. Most patients recovered from the paralysis which receded in the reverse of its onset. Some had respiratory weakness and abnormal heart rhythms. Landry called the disorder "acute ascending paralysis" which lead to the term Landry's Ascending Paralysis to describe the condition from then into the following century."[6]

"George Guillain, Jean Alexander Barré, and Andre Strohl, three French Army physicians, were tending to two paralyzed soldiers in 1916 when they determined to use a lumbar puncture, first used and described by Dr. Quinke

---

[4] Van den Berg, B. et al. Nature Review/Neurology 10, 2014, P. 472.

[5] Interview with Petra Williams, PT, PhD, Board Certified Neurologic Clinical Specialist and Assistant Professor, Northern Arizona University. June 2017.

[6] Goodfellow, John A. and Willison, Hugh J. "Guillain-Barré syndrome: a century of progress," Nature Reviews/Neurology, 2016, P. 1.

twenty-five years earlier. Samples of the patients' cerebrospinal fluid showed an abnormally high level of protein with a normal white cell count, distinguishing their paralysis from others, like syphilis and polio, where the white blood cells would also be highly elevated. This discovery separated Guillain-Barré Syndrome from other infective paralyses."[7]

IVIg and Plasmapheresis

One recommended therapy, plasmapheresis, was never used on me. "Therapeutic plasmapheresis or therapeutic plasma exchange (TPE) is a method for removing toxic elements from the blood. It is performed by removing blood, separating the plasma from the formed elements, and reinfusing the formed elements together with a plasma replacement."[8]

The other, Intravenous Immunoglobulin (IVIg), was used off and on throughout my hospital stay and during my early months at home. "IVIg is a blood product of highly concentrated globulin from thousands of healthy donors."[9] "It provides the patient with high concentrations of normal antibodies."[10] "Plasma exchange was the preferred treatment for GBS until a 1992 study proved IVIg to be as effective. With fewer side effects, IVIg has become the preferred treatment. In addition, it is easier to administer."[11]

"IVIg's method of action is less clear than that for plasmapheresis. Several mechanisms have been proposed, such as suppression of harmful white blood cells, supplying a large pool of naturally occurring and safe antibodies to neutralize harmful antibodies, blocking production of harmful antibodies, interference with the immune system's complement protein cascade that in GBS may cause nerve damage and inhibition of cytokines that attract myelin-

---

[7] Ibid, P. 1.

[8] "The Utility of Therapeutic Plasmapheresis for Neurological Disorders," NIH Consensus Development Conference Statement June 2-4, 1986. P. 1.

[9] Wu, Eveline, M.D. and Frank, Michael M., M.D., "The Mystery of IVIg," The Rheumatologist, March 8, 2012. P. 1.

[10] Guillain-Barré Syndrome, CIDP and Variants, GBS/CIDP Foundational International, 10th Edition (2010), P. 24.

[11] Meena, A.K., Khadilkar, S.V. and Murthy, J.M.K., "Treatment Guidelines for Guillain-Barré Syndrome," Annals of Indian Academy of Neurology, July, 2011. P. 6.

damaging macrophages."[12] While somewhat technical, this description explains why IVIg is used with GBS patients.

In Chapter Four

Pain in GBS

An article in Neurology: The Official Journal of the American Academy of Neurology states, "Pain in GBS may be pronounced and is often overlooked. (In our study) Pain was reported in the 2 weeks preceding weakness in 36% of patients, 66% reported pain in the acute phase...., and 38% reported pain after 1 year. In the majority of patients, the intensity of pain was moderate to severe. Longitudinal analysis showed high mean pain intensity scores during the entire follow-up. Pain occurred in the whole spectrum of GBS.....Only during later stages of disease, severity of weakness and disability were significantly correlated with intensity of pain." Conclusions of this study: "Pain is a common and often severe symptom of the whole spectrum of GBS. As it frequently occurs as the first symptom, but may even last for at least 1 year, pain in GBS requires full attention. It is likely that sensory nerve fiber involvement results in more severe pain."[13]

In Chapter Five

Ventilators and Respirators

The terms "respirator" and "ventilator" are often confused. A respirator is a mask-like device that filters fine particles from inhaled air. A ventilator is a machine that assists with or performs the breathing process for medical patients. The confusion is compounded because the specialists who assist a person on a ventilator are called respiratory therapists.

---

[12] Guillain-Barré Syndrome, CIDP and Variants, Ibid, P. 25.

[13] L. Ruts, PhD, MD, J. Drenthen, MD, J.L.M. Jongen, PhD, MD, W.C.J. Hop, PhD, G.H. Visser, PhD, MD, B.C. Jacobs, PhD, MD, P.A. van Doorn, PhD, MD, "Pain in Guillain-Barré syndrome: a long-term follow-up study," Neurology, The Official Journal of the American Academy of Neurology, September 22, 2010. P. 1.

In Chapter Six

Percutaneous Endoscopic Gastronomy (PEG)

"A percutaneous endoscopic gastrostomy (PEG) is a safe and effective way to provide food, liquids and medications directly into the stomach. The procedure is done for patients who are having trouble swallowing."[14] "Using a lighted, flexible tube called an endoscope, the physician creates a small opening from inside the stomach through the skin of the abdomen. A tube is secured to the abdomen wall with sutures. Nutrition is provided to the patient through the tube."[15]

Autonomic and Somatic Nervous Systems

"The somatic nervous system (SNS) is the part of the peripheral nervous system that handles voluntary control of body movements. It contains all the neurons connected with skeletal muscles and skin. Skeletal muscles are voluntary, and hence controlled by the somatic nervous system. They're one of the three major muscle groups, and are composed of muscles cells, all attached to bones by tendon fibers.

The autonomic nervous system (ANS) is the part of the peripheral nervous system that acts as an involuntary control system, below the level of consciousness, and controls visceral functions."[16]

"The autonomic nervous system controls the connections between the brain, spinal cord and organs/glands, whereas the SNS connects external sensory organs through the brain to the muscles."[17] "The ANS regulates fundamental states of physiology, including heart rate, digestion, respiratory rate, salivation,

---

[14] "Percutaneous Endoscopic Gastronomy," March 16, 2017, Cleveland Clinic website: (https://www.my.clevelandclinic.org/health/articles/percutaneous-endoscopic-gastronomy-peg) P. 1.
[15] Ibid.
[16] "Somatic and Autonomic Nervous Systems," Bethopedia, Psychology. (https://www.wiki.bethanycrane.com/somaticautonomousnervoussystems) P. 1.
[17] Ibid.

perspiration, pupillary dilation, energy utilization, temperature, and sexual arousal."[18]

In my case of GBS, the somatic nervous system was affected traumatically. Parts of the autonomic nervous system were also affected, particularly my heart rhythms and body temperature regulation.

Pain and Anxiety

"Even though paralyzed, (GBS) patients typically remain entirely lucid, and continue to feel pain and discomfort. The disease is psychologically dramatic, reducing the patient to profound physical and psychological helplessness with little warning. Such an experience may well be traumatic...."[19]

"Pain (in GBS) frequently occurs and may cause severe complaints. It often starts before the onset of weakness and therefore can lead to diagnostic difficulties."[20]

"The pain is often difficult to describe but tends to have an aching or cramping quality. There may be stabs of pain with movement. It is not at one clearly localized point but is somewhat diffuse and seems to be deep in the body rather than on the surface. It.....may be severe, particularly in patients with rapidly progressive and severe paralysis. In such patients, who may be on a ventilator and unable to communicate easily, it is very important to ask specifically if pain is present. (W)hen severe, it (the pain) may cause dangerous heart irregularities and changes in blood pressure and aggressive treatment with strong analgesics such as morphine may be needed.

(The physician author of this articles relates that) "It has been my experience that pain is frequently underappreciated and undertreated by physicians. Pain may occur during the acute phase of the illness and may even predate the onset of the weakness or it may occur during recovery and rehabilitation. (C)lose attention to anxiety and depression in both patients and their loved ones is a critical part of overall management of GBS."[21]

---

[18] Ibid, P. 2.

[19] "Post-Traumatic Stress Disorder as a Sequela of Guillain-Barré Syndrome," Journal of Traumatic Stress, Vol. 7, No. 4, 1994, P. 705

[20] Ibid.

[21] https://www.gbsnz.org.nz/.../Pain-in-the-Guillain-Barré-syndrome.doc. P. 1.

In Chapter Seven

Range of Motion

Range of Motion (ROM) is "The full movement potential of a joint, usually its range of flexion (bending) and extension."[22] "Muscle strength and flexibility are the key components to movement. Lack of activity due to injury or disease lead to a decline in these two vital functions. Range of motion helps maintain movement by stretching the muscles and moving the joints. There are active and passive range of motion. Active range of motion is exercises you do on your own. Passive means someone does the work for you."[23]

In Chapter Eight

Respiratory Therapists and the Suctioning Procedure

"The upper airway warms, cleans and moistens the air we breathe. The trach tube bypasses these mechanisms, so that the air moving through the tube is cooler, dryer and not as clean. In response to these changes, the body produces more mucus. "Suctioning," one of the responsibilities of respiratory therapists, "clears mucus from the tracheostomy tube and is essential for proper breathing. Also, secretions left in the tube could become contaminated and a chest infection could develop."[24]

"Suctioning is important to prevent a mucus plug from blocking the tube and stopping the patient's breathing. Suctioning should be considered:

- Any time the patient feels or hears mucus rattling in the tube or airway
- In the morning when the patient first wakes up
- When there is an increased respiratory rate (working hard to breathe)"[25]

---

[22] https://www.medicinenet.com/script/main/art.asp?articlekey=5208.

[23] Ferrara, Darla, "Active Vs Passive Range of Motion," at https://www.livestrong.com/article/339675-active-vs-passive-range-of-motion/ P. 1.

[24] Johns Hopkins Medicine (website), Tracheostomy Service, Suctioning, (https://www.hopkinsmedicine.org/tracheostomy/living/suctiong.html) P. 1

[25] Ibid, P. 2.

Because I could not alert the therapists when suctioning was necessary, they were more vigilant and suctioned my trach periodically throughout the day. Also, I was unaware that ".... suctioning too frequently" should be avoided[26] "as this could lead to more secretion buildup. They were trying to balance my need to be suctioned with the knowledge that too much suctioning could worsen the problem.

In Chapter Nine

Weaning from the Ventilator

"Discontinuation of mechanical ventilation is a two-step process, consisting of readiness testing and weaning:

> • Readiness testing – Readiness testing is the evaluation of objective criteria to determine whether a patient might be able to successfully and safely wean from mechanical ventilation.
> • Weaning – Weaning is the process of decreasing the amount of support that the patient receives from the mechanical ventilator, so the patient assumes a greater proportion of the ventilatory effort. The purpose is to assess the probability that mechanical ventilation can be successfully discontinued. Weaning may involve either an immediate shift from full ventilatory support to a period of breathing without assistance from the ventilator or a gradual reduction in the amount of ventilator support."[27]

"The Spontaneous Breathing Trial (SBT) is the traditional approach to weaning patients from mechanical ventilation.....As well as assessing whether a patient is ready for extubation (removal of the endotracheal tube), SBTs of increasing duration can be used to aid the weaning process and can be performed without disconnecting the patient from the ventilator."[28]

---

[26] Ibid, P. 2.

[27] Epstein, Scott K., MD, Walkey, Allan, MD. MSc. "Methods of weaning from mechanical ventilation." (https://www.uptodate.com/contents/methods-of-weaning-from-mechanical-ventilation) P. 1.

[28] Lermitte, Jeremy, BM FRCA and Garfield, Mark J., MB ChB FRCA. Weaning from mechanical ventilation. BJA, Volume 5, Issue 4, August 2005.

There are several variants of SBTs. "…. (these) include continuous positive airway pressure (CPAP)….and low-level pressure support ventilation (PSV) to overcome the resistance to breathing through an endotracheal tube…." When patients are considered ready to wean, the best way to assess whether they will breathe on their own is by undertaking an SBT. It has been demonstrated that by doing this the weaning process may be hastened.[29]

Passy-Muir Valve

"The Passy-Muir speaking valve is commonly used to help patients speak more normally. This one-way valve attaches to the outside opening of the tracheostomy tube and allows air to pass into the tracheostomy, but not out through it. The valve opens when the patient breathes in. When the patient breathes out, the valve closes and air flows around the tracheostomy tube, up through the vocal cords allowing sounds to be made. The patient breathes out through the mouth and nose instead of the tracheostomy."[30]

"Some patients may immediately adjust to breathing with the valve in place. Others may need to gradually increase the time the valve is worn. Breathing out with the valve (around the tracheostomy tube) is harder work than breathing out through the tracheostomy tube. Patients may need to build up the strength and ability to use the valve, but most children will be able to use the speaking valve all day after a period of adjustment."[31]

In Chapter Eleven

Anxiety and Depression

"Psychiatric symptoms are common among persons with GBS and tend to develop during the period of acute care. These may include emotional

---

(https://www.academic.oup.com/bjaed/article/5/4/113/475175/Weaning-from-mechanical-ventilation) P.1.
[29] Ibid.
[30] "Tracheostomy and Passy-Muir Valve,"
https://www.johnshopkinsmedicine.org/tracheostomy/living/passey-muir_valve.html P. 1.
[31] Ibid.

disturbances, feelings of hopelessness, and demoralization."[32] Weiss et al, in a 2002 study of 49 severely compromised GBS patients, found 82% expressed anxiety, 67% had depressive symptoms, and 20% expressed hopelessness. Such symptoms occurred independently, in combination, or as features of a subacute confusional state. At the conclusion of ICU care, 35% of GBS patients continue to experience long-lasting distress, and 18% experience continued anxiety.[33]

"Pain management, effective communication, assistive devices, and treatment with antidepressants may be helpful in the management of psychiatric symptoms during recovery from GBS."[34]

In Chapter Twelve

Axonal Damage

In 1986 an axonal type of GBS was identified. Rather than attacking solely the myelin sheath covering the nerves, in this variant the axons are also attacked. (Axons are long fiber-like structures extending from a cell body.)

Thousands of axons bundled together form a nerve. The axon conducts nerve impulses away from the nerve body.[35]

"In the 1990s, a pure motor axonal form of GBS, designated acute motor axonal neuropathy (AMAN), was recognized in northern China and later reported in other countries."[36] Dr. M recorded in my medical record his concern that I might have the AMAN variant of GBS.

---

[32] Brousseau, Kristin; Arciniegas, David; Harris, Susan. "Pharmacologic management of anxiety and affective lability during recovery from Guillain-Barré Syndrome: some preliminary observations. Neuropsychiatric Disease and Treatment. US National Library of Medicine. National Institutes of Health. P1.

[33] Ibid.

[34] Ibid.

[35] Hiraga, A; Mon, M; Ogawara, K; Kojima, S; Kanesaka, T; Misawa, S; Hatton, T; Kuwabara, S. "Recovery patterns and long-term prognosis for axonal Guillain-Barré Syndrome," Journal of Neurology, Neurosurgery & Psychiatry. Vol. 76, issue 5. P. 719.

[36] Ibid.

In Chapter Fourteen

Electromyography

"Electromyography .... attempts to pinpoint what is affecting a patient's muscles and nerves. The test, which usually takes 30-60 minutes, requires a physician to insert electrode needles into the muscles to monitor and record their electrical activity.... The activity recorded from the needles is projected on a screen that requires the specialist to interpret the readings as they are being transmitted."[37]

"Another part of the EMG test is the nerve conduction study that examines both the size (amplitude) of the responses from muscles and sensory nerves and the speed (conduction velocity) that it takes for the nerves to transmit the signal. The findings on nerve conduction testing are important in diagnosing the various forms of peripheral neuropathy .... (including) Guillain-Barré Syndrome ...."[38]

---

[37] Cedars-Sinai website (https://www.cedars-sinai.edu/Patients/Programs-and-Services/Neurology/Centers-and-Programs/Neuromuscular-Disorders/Precise-Diagnostics-Lead-to-Superior-Care.aspx)
[38] Ibid.

Acknowledgments

Writing a book about our battle with Guillain-Barré Syndrome would never have occurred without gentle pressure and constant encouragement from our son Eric who, knowing the power of the written word, anticipated its benefit for healthcare providers and patients. Physical therapy students at Ohio University and Northern Arizona University spurred the writing with enthusiastic endorsement of the messages I conveyed in my lectures about the challenges of recovering from this disease as well as therapists' role in achieving that goal. Numerous friends pushed, usually with quiet insistence assuring us it would be worth the effort. I am grateful to Steve Loebs and Bernie Zahern for making sure I never gave up on this project.

The manuscript benefitted immensely from readers and editors who took so much time to offer critiques, corrections, observations, and bold editing. My appreciation to Jim Breiner, Barbara Brandt, Carolyn Roberts, Karen Snyder, Sylvia White, Karl Stoerker, Ned Yellig, Karen Mueller, Robert Petrella, Seth Oberst, Emile Bareng, Elizabeth Huls, Sandra Cornett, Petra Williams and most especially to Eric who made sure we cut out about a third of the rambling narrative.

Special thanks to Owen Lowery who captured so brilliantly both my utter despair as well as eternal hope for full recovery in his artful cover design.

In a last word, this book could not have been written without Stu's and my passage through the agony of Guillain-Barré Syndrome. During that journey many health professionals contributed to my recovery. While all cannot be named here, I hope they will recognize themselves in the narrative and know my heartfelt gratitude. Petra is an exception. With her knowledge of physical therapy techniques and her determination, she helped my body recover and, in the end, saved my total being.

And for the hundreds of friends and relatives who supported both Stu and me during this long ordeal, know that all the kindnesses you offered contributed immeasurably to our recovery. Sandy Harbrecht, especially, went far beyond what any employer would do by saving my job, visiting me throughout my long hospital stay, and remaining, always, a true friend.

Bonnie, Glen, Katie, and Eric: there is no way we could have survived without you.

Made in the USA
Middletown, DE
03 May 2022

65179766R00102